Contents

W0227863

Guide to Assessment Scales in Parkinson's Disease

Pablo Martinez-Martin

Research Unit, Alzheimer Centre Reina Sofia Foundation and Centre for Networked Biomedical Research on Neurodegenerative Diseases (CIBERNED), Carlos III Institute of Health, Madrid, Spain

Carmen Rodriguez-Blazquez

Area of Applied Epidemiology, National Centre for Epidemiology and Centre for Networked Biomedical Research on Neurodegenerative Diseases (CIBERNED), Carlos III Institute of Health, Madrid, Spain

Maria João Forjaz

National School of Public Health and REDISSEC, Carlos III Institute of Health, Madrid, Spain

Kallol Ray Chaudhuri

National Parkinson Foundation International Centre of Excellence, King's College London, London, United Kingdom

King's Neuroscience Research and Development, King's College Hospital and University Hospital Lewisham, London, United Kingdom

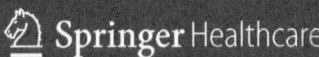

Published by Springer Healthcare Ltd, 236 Gray's Inn Road, London, WC1X 8HB, UK.

www.springerhealthcare.com

© 2014 Springer Healthcare, a part of Springer Science+Business Media.

British Library Cataloguing-in-Publication Data.

A catalogue record for this book is available from the British Library.

ISBN 978-1-907673-87-0

Although every effort has been made to ensure that drug doses and other information are presented accurately in this publication, the ultimate responsibility rests with the prescribing physician. Neither the publisher nor the authors can be held responsible for errors or for any consequences arising from the use of the information contained herein. Any product mentioned in this publication should be used in accordance with the prescribing information prepared by the manufacturers. No claims or endorsements are made for any drug or compound at present under clinical investigation.

Project editor: Nicola Cartridge and Katrina Dorn
Designer: Joe Harvey
Production: Marina Maher
Printed in Great Britain by Latimer Trend

Author biographies

Pablo Martínez-Martín is a graduate in Medicine, and Neurology, and a tenured scientist for the Spanish Public Boards of Research. Since 2006, he has served as the Scientific Director of the Research Unit for Alzheimer's Disease, CIEN Foundation, the Alzheimer Centre Reina Sofía Foundation, and a member of the Consortium for Biomedical Research in Neurodegenerative Diseases (CIBERNED), Carlos III Institute of Health (Spanish Ministry of Economy and Competitiveness). Dr Martinez-Martin's research interests are: clinical assessment and rating scales; patient-reported outcomes, particularly health-related quality of life; neurodegenerative diseases; Parkinson's disease; and Alzheimer's disease and dementia. He has received 14 awards for scientific activities in neurosciences and aging. Dr. Martínez-Martín has authored over 290 articles in peer-reviewed scientific journals and 87 book chapters, and is editor or co-editor of 17 books and monographs. He has participated in 348 platform or poster reports and 168 talks in scientific forums (congresses, symposia, expert workshops) and has given 159 lectures as invited professor in teaching institutions. At present, he is an active member of several study groups with the Spanish Society of Neurology and the Movement Disorder Society, as well as international steering committees for research and collaborative groups.

Carmen Rodríguez-Blázquez is a psychologist (National University of Distance Education, UNED) and research assistant at the National Centre of Epidemiology (Carlos III Institute of Health), where she participates in several national and international research projects on clinical and social aspects of neurological diseases (such as Parkinson's and Alzheimer's diseases), quality of life of older populations, and questionnaire adaptation and validation. She has also authored more than 30 papers in peer-reviewed scientific journals and book chapters on the field of disabilities, neurological diseases, quality of life, and psychometric properties of scales and questionnaires. She has participated in the translation and validation of the Spanish official version of the Movement Disorders Society-Unified Parkinson's Disease Rating Scale (MDS-UPDRS).

Maria João Forjaz is a scientific researcher at National School of Public Health, at the Spanish National School of Public Health; Carlos III Institute of Health. She graduated from the University of Lisbon and in 2000, as a Fulbright scholar, obtained her doctorate in clinical psychology from the University of North Texas, USA. Her main research interests are quality of life in Parkinson's disease and older adults, assessment of non-motor symptoms, and scale validation using classic psychometric and Rasch analysis techniques. She is the principal investigator of several research grants on the quality of life of older adults and she combines her research activity with teaching and tutoring Master in Public Health students. She is a member of the Spanish Research Network on Health Services and Chronicity (REDISSEC), where she collaborates with research on patient-reported outcome measures and the impact of comorbidity and the functional ability of older adults. She is also a member of the Movement Disorders Society Tremor Task Force. Dr. Forjaz is the author of over 40 articles in peer-review journal as well as several book chapters.

Kallol Ray Chaudhuri is a Professor of neurology and movement disorders and consultant neurologist at the King's College London Institute of Psychiatry and a principal investigator at the Medical Research Council Centre for Neurodegeneration Research at King's College London. He is also the medical director of the National Parkinson Foundation International Centre of Excellence at King's College, London. He sits on the Nervous Systems Committee of the UK Department of Health, National Institute of Health Research and also serves as co-chairman of the appointments/liaison committee of the Movement Disorders Society (MDS), where he is currently serving as the member of the scientific programme committee. He is the Chairman of the MDS non-motor study group and is on the scientific program committee for the MDS Congress (2013–2015). He serves on the American Academy of Neurology Practice Parameter task force for Parkinson's disease (PD), restless legs syndrome (RLS), and more recently, non-motor symptoms in PD. He is the European Editor of *Basal Ganglia* and is on the editorial board of *Parkinsonism and Related Disorders* and *Journal of Parkinson's Disease*. He is also the lead for London South Comprehensive Local Research Network neurosciences sub-speciality group. Professor Chaudhuri is the author of 227 papers, including reviews and book chapters, is co-editor of 4 books on PD and RLS, and has published over 200 peer-reviewed abstracts. He is the chief editor of the first comprehensive textbook on non motor aspects of PD, published by Oxford University Press, and is recipient of the British Medical Association book commendation prize. He has contributed extensively to educational radio and television interviews, including BBC and CNN, newspaper articles, and videos. He has also lectured extensively on PD and RLS at international meetings in USA, Japan, Europe, South America, South Africa, India, and Australia. His major research interests are continuous drug delivery treatment of PD and restless legs syndrome, Parkisnonism in minority ethnic groups, and sleep problems in PD. In 2005, he was awarded a DSc degree by the University of London.

1. Introduction

Importance of assessment scales in Parkinson's disease

To 'measure' entails the quantification of something by comparison with a fixed magnitude of the same species taken as the unit. This way, the attribute to be measured must be directly observable and a unit has to exist (eg, physical measures). However, many human attributes (eg, intelligence and emotions) are not observable and lack a unit of measurement. These conceptual or abstract objects are named 'constructs'.

The use of scales for assessment in neurology arises from the need to quantify disorders and states (such constructs as disability, symptoms, quality of life) for which genuine measures do not exist and to obtain pragmatic and comprehensive information that cannot be procured from available 'objective' methods (due to costs, need of equipment and expert personnel, conditions of application, etc.).

Initially, rating scales for Parkinson's disease (PD) were designed by an expert or group of experts and used with minimal or no previous testing of their quality as measurement instruments. This situation was characterized by a great variability in the design, content, and metric quality of available scales, resulting in a lack of comparability between studies using these tools. At present, however, systematic application of standardized methods for development, analysis, and formal testing of health status measures for PD is increasingly used.

This guide intends to summarize the characteristics of relevant rating scales and questionnaires for PD. Most of the included instruments, generic or specific for PD, have been qualified as 'recommended' by the ad hoc Movement Disorder Society Task Force (www.movementdisorders.org/publications/ebm_reviews/) and the template for presentation of data is based on the different models used by this task force. Data on the properties of each measure and recognized standard values for comparison are also shown. Recommended references for interested readers appear at the end of each section.

Classification

Scales used to assess PD may be classified into two categories: generic (ie, those scales usable in any health condition), and specific (ie, scales developed for exclusive use in PD). Also, they may be classified as single-item, multi-item or composite scale; unidimensional or multidimensional; and as disease or patient-centered measures. Disease-centered scales reflect aspects of interest to clinicians, such as severity and signs of the disease, disability, and motor complication, whereas patient-centered measures assess the impact of the disease from a patient's perspective and are linked to quality of life and psychosocial adjustment.

© Springer Healthcare 2014
P. Martinez-Martin et al., *Guide to Assessment Scales in Parkinson's Disease,*
DOI: 10.1007/978-1-907673-88-7_1

Design and validation of scales

The creation and validation of a rating scale is a complex task. Most areas relevant to the goal being pursued should be identified and included; the scale components must be specifically related to such areas and provide scores suitable for statistical analysis. Importantly, the scale should be as simple and as brief as possible. The first version of the measure is applied to a relatively small number of individuals from the target population in a pilot study aimed at identifying flaws and ambiguities. In addition, pilot studies provide preliminary data on acceptability and reliability, and allows shortening of the scale when necessary.

The definitive version of the scale is obtained through revision and refinement following these pilot studies. This version must be validated in a representative sample of the target population through a new study to determine the quality of the scale. Principles for rating scales validation come from the Classical Test Theory and Modern Test Theory, including Item Response Theory, and Rasch analysis [1–4].

Attributes and criteria of the rating scales

In the process of validation the following attributes should be tested to ascertain whether a scale is an effective instrument of measurement [1,5–7].

Conceptual model - rationale for and description of the concept and populations that the measure intends to assess.

Acceptability – refers to how acceptable an instrument is for respondents to complete and the extent to which the scores are well distributed in the sample.

Dimensionality – refers to the grouping of items in domains or latent variables.

Scaling assumptions – equivalence of the items in distribution of response options, and how correctly the items are grouped into scales**.**

Reliability – extent to which the scale is free of random error. Two aspects are distinguishable in this section: internal consistency (interrelation among scale components at a point in time) and reproducibility or stability of scores among different raters (inter-rater reliability) and at different moments of time (intra-rater or test-retest reliability).

Validity – ability of the scale to measure what it purports to measure. Content validity refers to the extent to which the construct of interest is adequately sampled by the scale components (items, questions). Criterion-related validity refers to the relationship between the scale and a gold standard (the 'criterion'), although there is no gold standard available for most of the constructs measured in neurology or movement disorders. Construct validity refers to the evidence that supports an interpretation of the scores based on the theoretical framework related to the construct being measured (hypotheses-testing). Within the construct validity, convergent validity refers to the relations of the scale with other measures for the same construct, while divergent validity refers to the absence of relations with measures for constructs different to the one being measured. Discriminative validity (known-groups or extreme-groups validity) represents the measure's ability to detect differences among specific groups in a single observation.

Precision (sensitivity) – refers to the ability of a scale to distinguish between small differences.
Responsiveness – related to precision, it refers to the ability of the scale to detect changes over time.

Interpretability – degree to which a comprehensible meaning can be assigned to the scale scores.
Other related aspects – respondent and administrative burden; alternative forms (different modes of administration: phone, interview, self-assessment); and cross-cultural adaptation (translation and adaptation to obtain an equivalent linguistic and conceptual version to be used in a different language or culture than the original).

Most of these measurement properties are analyzed using statistical methods and standard values or 'criteria' of quality have been proposed for the results (examples are shown in Table 1.1). Before using a scale in clinical practice or research, most of these criteria must be verified.

Table 1.1 Standard values for basic attributes of scales

Attribute	Value	Reference
Feasibility		
Missing data	<5%	[8]
Acceptability		
Floor and ceiling effects	<15%	[9]
Skewness	−1 to +1	[10]
Internal consistency		
Cronbach's alpha	α>0.70 (group); 0.90–0.95 (individual)	[6]
Inter-item correlation	r>0.20 and r<0.75	[8]
Item-total correlation	r>0.20 – r>0.40	[5,11]
Homogeneity coefficient	r>0.30	[12]
Reliability		
Inter-observer – nominal or ordinal	*Kappa* r>0.60 or r>0.70	[13]
Continuous data	Intraclass correlation coefficient r>0.70	[7]
Test-retest – nominal or ordinal	*Kappa* r>0.60 or r>0.70	
Continuous data	Intraclass correlation coefficient r>0.70	
Construct validity (Hypotheses-testing)		
Convergent validity	r>0.40 – r>0.60	[14,15]
Divergent validity	r<0.30	
Internal validity	r=0.30–0.70	[16]
Known-groups validity	Significant difference between groups	[17]

The guide: intention and organization

The review of scales presented in this Guide has been systematically adapted to these clinimetric attributes, following the proforma shown as Table 1.2. Our intention is to provide rapid and pragmatic information on the relevant aspects related to the characteristics and clinimetric properties of the most relevant scales used in PD.

Table 1.2 Guide to Assessment Scales in Parkingson's Disease

Scale Original reference	
Description of scale	Construct to be measured
	Content: number of items and subscales, answer options, type of scoring
	Time to complete the scale
	Time frame
	Rater: Patient /proxy, care professional…
	Generic/specific
Copyright?	Copyright or public domain?
How can the scale be obtained	How to access the scale
Clinimetric properties of the scale in patients with PD	
Feasibility	Appropriateness of questions for PD population
	Applicability across PD stages: mild, moderate, severe?
Dimensionality	The number of domains or dimensions that compose the scale
Acceptability	Floor and ceiling effects
	Score distribution
Reliability	Internal consistency
	Inter-rater reliability
	Test-retest reliability
Validity	Face/content validity
	Construct validity (convergent, known-groups, internal)
	Any other types of validity (eg, predictive)
	Scale validity tested for PD in different cultural settings?
Responsiveness & Interpretability	Sensitive to changes in the construct?
	Minimal clinically important change ?
	Scale valid for people with PD of both genders and at all ages?
Cross-cultural adaptations & Others	Translations & adaptations
Overall impression	
Advantages and disadvantages	List of advantages
	List of disadvantages

Selected scales are included in the guide. Owing to copyright restrictions of some of the instruments, this was not permitted for all of the rating scales. However, in all cases, a source from where the scale can be obtained is provided.

References

1 Nunnally JC, Bernstein IH. *Psychometric Theory*. New York: McGraw Hill; 1994.

2 DeVellis RF. Classical test theory. *Med Care*. 2006;44(suppl 3):S50-559.

3 Hays RD, Morales LS, Reise SP. Item response theory and health outcomes measurement in the 21st century. *Med Care*. 2000;38(suppl 9):II28-42.

4 Andrich D. Rating scales and Rasch measurement. *Expert Rev Pharmacoecon Outcomes Res*. 2011;1:571-585.

5 Streiner DL, Norman GR. Selecting the items. In: *Health measurement scales. A practical guide to their development and use*. 4th edn. Oxford: Oxford University Press; 2008: 87.

6 Aaronson N, Alonso J, Burnam A, et al. Assessing health status and quality-of-life instruments: attributes and review criteria. *Qual Life Res*. 2002;11:193-205.

7 Terwee CB, Bot SDM, De Boer MR, et al. Quality criteria were proposed for measurement properties of health status questionnaires. *J Clin Epidemiol*. 2007;60:34-42.

8 Smith SC, Lamping DL, Banerjee S, et al. Measurement of health-related quality of life for people with dementia: development of a new instrument (DEMQOL) and an evaluation of current methodology. *Health Technol Assess*. 2005;9:1-93.

9 McHorney CA, Tarlov AR. Individual-patient monitoring in clinical practice: are available health status surveys adequate? *Qual Life Res*. 1995;4:293-307.

10 van der Linden FA, Kragt JJ, Klein M, van der Ploeg HM, Polman CH, Uitdehaag BMJ. Psychometric evaluation of the multiple sclerosis impact scale (MSIS-29) for proxy use. *J Neurol Neurosurg Psychiatr*. 2005;76:1677-1681.

11 Ware JE Jr, Gandek B. Methods for testing data quality, scaling assumptions, and reliability: the IQOLA Project approach. International Quality of Life Assessment. *J Clin Epidemiol*. 1998;51:945-952.

12 Eisen M, Ware JE, Donald CA, Brook RH. Measuring components of children's health status. *Med Care*. 1979;17:902-921.

13 Landis JR, Koch GG. The measurement of observer agreement for categorical data. *Biometrics*. 1977;33:159-174.

14 Chassany O, Sagnier P, Marquis P, Fullerton S, Aaronson N. Patient-reported outcomes: the example of health-related quality of life—a European guidance document for the improved integration of health-related quality of life assessment in the drug regulatory process. *Drug Inf J*. 2002;36:209-238.

15 Fitzpatrick R, Davey C, Buxton MJ, Jones DR. Evaluating patient-based outcome measures for use in clinical trials. *Health Technol Assess*. 1998;2:1-74.

16 Hobart J, Lamping D, Fitzpatrick R, Riazi A, Thompson A. The Multiple Sclerosis Impact Scale (MSIS-29): a new patient-based outcome measure. *Brain*. 2001;124(Part 5):962-973.

17 Fayers P, Machin D. Developing a questionnaire. In: *Quality of Life*. Chichester: Wiley; 2000:51.

2. Multi-domain scales

The complex nature of Parkinson's disease (PD) requires the use of multi-purpose and comprehensive assessment tools that cover a wide array of symptoms. The Unified Parkinson's Disease Rating Scale (UPDRS) has been widely used and extensively tested for its clinimetric properties. The recently developed Movement Disorders Society (MDS) sponsored revision of the Unified Parkinson's Disease Rating Scale (MDS-UPDRS) has shown satisfactory quality of its attributes and probably will replace the UPDRS in the coming years.

Unified Parkinson's Disease Rating Scale (UPDRS) (Figure 2.1) [1]	
Description of scale	
Overview	The UPDRS assesses PD-related disability and impairment [2]
	Composed of 42 items grouped into four subscales:
	I, Mentation, Behavior and Mood (4 items);
	II, Activities of Daily Living (ADL) (13 items);
	III, Motor (14 items, 27 scores);
	IV, Complications of Therapy (11 items). It also includes the modified Hoehn & Yahr Staging Scale (HY) and the Schwab & England Activities of Daily Living Scale (SE)
	In subscales I to III, items are scored on a four-point scale. In subscale IV, some items are dichotomous and others are scored on a four-point scale for duration or severity
	Time for administration: 10 to 20 minutes
	Time frame: time of assessment or past week (for Section IV)
	Rated by the health professionals. Sections I and II can be self-administered [3,4]
	Specific for PD
Copyright?	Public domain
How can the scale be obtained?	The scale can be obtained from the original publication [1]
Clinimetric properties of scale in patients with PD	
Feasibility	Used in all stages of PD, but the scale favors the assessment of moderate and severe impairments. Floor effect limits the scale's utility in early stages of PD
Dimensionality	Multitrait scaling and factor analysis have revealed four factors, each one corresponding to a subscale [5]. Factor structure of the Motor section has been analyzed [5–7]

© Springer Healthcare 2014

P. Martinez-Martin et al., *Guide to Assessment Scales in Parkinson's Disease*,
DOI: 10.1007/978-1-907673-88-7_2

Acceptability	Observed scores coincided with the possible score ranges only in Section III [5]
	Floor effect in Sections I and IV [2,5]
Reliability	Cronbach's alpha ranged from 0.64 (Section I) to 0.92 (Sections II and III) [5,8]. ADL and Motor sections can be reduced to eight items each without losing reliability or validity [9]
	Inter-rater reliability is adequate for the total UPDRS and for Sections II and III [2]
	Test-retest reliability is acceptable; higher for early-stage PD [4,5,10]
Validity	Face/content validity has been considered adequate only for Motor Examination [11]
	Correlations with other PD scales: UPDRS Mentation and Complications with HY, moderate; UPDRS ADL and Motor Exam with SE, high correlation [11]
	Known-groups validity: significantly different UPDRS subscales scores by HY stages [11]
Responsiveness & Interpretability	Standard error of measurement (SEM) ranged from 1.24 (UPDRS Mentation) to 2.48 (UPDRS Motor) [5]
	UPDRS is responsive to therapeutic interventions and is the reference scale for regulatory agencies. Minimally detectable change (MDC) ranged from 2 (Mentation) to 11 (Motor Examination). MDC for total score was 13 [8]. Minimal clinically relevant incremental difference (MCRID) was established in a range from 4 to 10 points for UPDRS Motor [2]
	The effects of sex and age on UPDRS ratings during treatment interventions have not been specifically examined [2]
Cross-cultural Adaptations & Others	Translated and validated into many languages. Alternative ways of administration for self, caregivers and nursing staff assessments have been tested [3,12]
Overall impression	
Advantages	Uniformity of communication; teaching tapes available through the MDS [13]
Disadvantages	Excessive length; redundancies in ADL and Motor sections [14]; insufficient items to assess non-motor symptoms of PD; lack of standardized instructions; different score system in Section IV; inconsistent allocation of items to specific sections; cultural bias

Movement Disorders Society sponsored revision of the Unified Parkinson's Disease Rating Scale (MDS-UPDRS) [15]	
Description of scale	
Overview	Assesses the motor and non-motor impact of PD
	Part I: Non-Motor Experiences of Daily Living, with six rater-based items and seven for self-assessment; Part II: Motor Experiences of Daily Living, with 13 patient-based items; Part III: Motor Examination (33 scores based on 18 items, due to left, right and other body distributions); and Part IV: Motor Complications, with six items [15]
	Rating for items: 0 (normal) to 4 (severe). Total score for each Part is obtained from the sum of the corresponding item scores
	Time estimated: 30 minutes for the full scale, 10 minutes for Part III
	Time frame: the past week for Parts I, II, and IV. Time of assessment for Part III
	Specific for PD
Copyright?	Owned by the MDS
How can the scale be obtained?	www.movementdisorders.org/publications/rating_scales
Clinimetric properties of scale in patients with PD	
Feasibility	Specifically designed for patients with PD. Vocabulary avoids medical jargon and is adapted to a seventh-grade level [15]
	Designed to be applicable to patients with PD across various levels of disabilities [16]. Scores significantly increase with disease duration and HY stages [17]
Dimensionality	Multidimensional scale, with four sections [15,18,19]
Acceptability	Mild/moderate floor effect present in Part IV. No ceiling effect. [15]
Reliability	Cronbach's alpha: from 0.79 (Part I) to 0.93 (Part III) [15,19,20]
	Inter-rater reliability: not tested
	Test-retest reliability: satisfactory in the Spanish validation [19]
Validity	Content validity: evaluated during the scale development phase [16]; not formally tested
	Convergent validity: strongly correlated with UPDRS [15]. HY showed moderate correlations with Parts I and IV, and high correlations with Parts II and III. Clinical Impression of Severity Index for Parkinson's Disease (CISI-PD) showed high correlations with all MDS-UPDRS sections [17-19]. As a whole, Part I items showed moderate-to-high correlations with scales assessing similar constructs [20,21]
	Known-groups: MDS-UPDRS scores significantly increased with age (Parts I and III), disease duration, years of treatment, and HY stages [17,19]
	Internal validity: moderate to high correlation between the subscales [16,19]
Responsiveness & Interpretability	Responsive to therapeutic interventions [22–24], although its use in clinical trials is still scarce
	Scores from UPDRS and other scales can be converted into MDS-UPDRS respective scores (and vice-versa) using equation models [21,25,26]

Cross-cultural Adaptations & Others	Translations into several languages are available in the MDS website (see above). More translations are ongoing through the MDS-UPDRS translation program [27]
Overall impression	
Advantages	Satisfactory clinimetric properties; translation and cross-cultural adaptation program; certificate training program available through the MDS [28]
Disadvantages	Length (50 items; 65 scores). Responsiveness not tested

Figure 2.1 Unified Parkinson's Disease Rating Scale (UPDRS)

I. Mentation, Behavior And Mood

1. Intellectual Impairment

0 = None.

1 = Mild. Consistent forgetfulness with partial recollection of events and no other difficulties.

2 = Moderate memory loss, with disorientation and moderate difficulty handling complex problems. Mild but definite impairment of function at home with need of occasional prompting.

3 = Severe memory loss with disorientation for time and often to place. Severe impairment in handling problems.

4 = Severe memory loss with orientation preserved to person only. Unable to make judgements or solve problems. Requires much help with personal care. Cannot be left alone at all.

2. Thought disorder (Due to dementia or drug intoxication)

0 = None.

1 = Vivid dreaming.

2 = "Benign" hallucinations with insight retained.

3 = Occasional to frequent hallucinations or delusions; without insight; could interfere with daily activities.

4 = Persistent hallucinations, delusions, or florrid psychosis. Not able to care for self.

3. Depression

1 = Periods of sadness or guilt greater than normal, never sustained for days or weeks.

2 = Sustained depression (1 week or more).

3 = Sustained depression with vegetative symptoms (insomnia, anorexia, weight loss, loss of interest).

4 = Sustained depression with vegetative symptoms and suicidal thoughts or intent.

4. Motivation/Initiative

0 = Normal.

1 = Less assertive than usual; more passive.

2 = Loss of initiative or disinterest in elective (nonroutine) activities.

3 = Loss of initiative or disinterest in day to day (routine) activities.

4 = Withdrawn, complete loss of motivation.

II. Activities of daily living (for both "on" and "off")

5. Speech

0 = Normal.

1 = Mildly affected. No difficulty being understood.

2 = Moderately affected. Sometimes asked to repeat statements.

3 = Severely affected. Frequently asked to repeat statements.

4 = Unintelligible most of the time.

6. *Salivation*
0 = Normal.
1 = Slight but definite excess of saliva in mouth; may have nighttime drooling.
2 = Moderately excessive saliva; may have minimal drooling.
3 = Marked excess of saliva with some drooling.
4 = Marked drooling, requires constant tissue or handkerchief.

7. *Swallowing*
0 = Normal.
1 = Rare choking.
2 = Occasional choking.
3 = Requires soft food.
4 = Requires NG tube or gastrotomy feeding.

8. *Handwriting*
0 = Normal.
1 = Slightly slow or small.
2 = Moderately slow or small; all words are legible.
3 = Severely affected; not all words are legible.
4 = The majority of words are not legible.

9. *Cutting food and handling utensils*
0 = Normal.
1 = Somewhat slow and clumsy, but no help needed.
2 = Can cut most foods, although clumsy and slow; some help needed.
3 = Food must be cut by someone, but can still feed slowly.
4 = Needs to be fed.

10. *Dressing*
0 = Normal.
1 = Somewhat slow, but no help needed.
2 = Occasional assistance with buttoning, getting arms in sleeves.
3 = Considerable help required, but can do some things alone.
4 = Helpless.

11. *Hygiene*
0 = Normal.
1 = Somewhat slow, but no help needed.
2 = Needs help to shower or bathe; or very slow in hygienic care.
3 = Requires assistance for washing, brushing teeth, combing hair, going to bathroom.
4 = Foley catheter or other mechanical aids.

12. *Turning in bed and adjusting bed clothes*
0 = Normal.
1 = Somewhat slow and clumsy, but no help needed.
2 = Can turn alone or adjust sheets, but with great difficulty.
3 = Can initiate, but not turn or adjust sheets alone.
4 = Helpless.

13. Falling (unrelated to freezing)
0 = None.
1 = Rare falling.
2 = Occasionally falls, less than once per day.
3 = Falls an average of once daily.
4 = Falls more than once daily.

14. Freezing when walking
0 = None.
1 = Rare freezing when walking; may have starthesitation.
2 = Occasional freezing when walking.
3 = Frequent freezing. Occasionally falls from freezing.
4 = Frequent falls from freezing.

15. Walking
0 = Normal.
1 = Mild difficulty. May not swing arms or may tend to drag leg.
2 = Moderate difficulty, but requires little or no assistance.
3 = Severe disturbance of walking, requiring assistance.
4 = Cannot walk at all, even with assistance.

16. Tremor (symptomatic complaint of tremor in any part of body.)
0 = Absent.
1 = Slight and infrequently present.
2 = Moderate; bothersome to patient.
3 = Severe; interferes with many activities.
4 = Marked; interferes with most activities.

17. Sensory complaints related to parkinsonism
0 = None.
1 = Occasionally has numbness, tingling, or mild aching.
2 = Frequently has numbness, tingling, or aching; not distressing.
3 = Frequent painful sensations.
4 = Excruciating pain.

III. Motor Examination
18. Speech
0 = Normal.
1 = Slight loss of expression, diction and/or volume.
2 = Monotone, slurred but understandable; moderately impaired.
3 = Marked impairment, difficult to understand.
4 = Unintelligible.

19. Facial expression
0 = Normal.
1 = Minimal hypomimia, could be normal "Poker Face".
2 = Slight but definitely abnormal diminution of facial expression
3 = Moderate hypomimia; lips parted some of the time.
4 = Masked or fixed facies with severe or complete loss of facial expression; lips parted 1/4 inch or more.
   (head, upper and lower extremities)

20. *Tremor at rest*
0 = Absent.
1 = Slight and infrequently present.
2 = Mild in amplitude and persistent. Or moderate in amplitude, but only intermittently present.
3 = Moderate in amplitude and present most of the time.
4 = Marked in amplitude and present most of the time.

21. *Action or Postural Tremor of hands*
0 = Absent.
1 = Slight; present with action.
2 = Moderate in amplitude, present with action.
3 = Moderate in amplitude with posture holding as well as action.
4 = Marked in amplitude; interferes with feeding.

22. *Rigidity (Judged on passive movement of major joints with patient relaxed in sitting position. Cogwheeling to be ignored.)*
0 = Absent.
1 = Slight or detectable only when activated by mirror or other movements.
2 = Mild to moderate.
3 = Marked, but full range of motion easily achieved.
4 = Severe, range of motion achieved with difficulty.

23. *Finger taps* (Patient taps thumb with index finger in rapid succession.)
0 = Normal.
1 = Mild slowing and/or reduction in amplitude.
2 = Moderately impaired. Definite and early fatiguing. May have occasional arrests in movement.
3 = Severely impaired. Frequent hesitation in initiating movements or arrests in ongoing movement.
4 = Can barely perform the task.

24. *Hand movements* (patient opens and closes hands in rapid succesion.)
0 = Normal.
1 = Mild slowing and/or reduction in amplitude.
2 = Moderately impaired. Definite and early fatiguing. May have occasional arrests in movement.
3 = Severely impaired. Frequent hesitation in initiating movements or arrests in ongoing movement.
4 = Can barely perform the task.

25. *Rapid alternating movements of hands* (pronation-supination movements of hands, vertically and horizontally, with as large an amplitude as possible, both hands simultaneously.)
0 = Normal.
1 = Mild slowing and/or reduction in amplitude.
2 = Moderately impaired. Definite and early fatiguing. May have occasional arrests in movement.
3 = Severely impaired. Frequent hesitation in initiating movements or arrests in ongoing movement.
4 = Can barely perform the task.

26. *Leg agility* (patient taps heel on the ground in rapid succession picking up entire leg. Amplitude should be at least 3 inches.)
0 = Normal.
1 = Mild slowing and/or reduction in amplitude.
2 = Moderately impaired. Definite and early fatiguing. May have occasional arrests in movement.
3 = Severely impaired. Frequent hesitation in initiating movements or arrests in ongoing movement.
4 = Can barely perform the task.

27. *Arising from chair* (patient attempts to rise from a straightbacked chair, with arms folded across chest.)
0 = Normal.
1 = Slow; or may need more than one attempt.
2 = Pushes self up from arms of seat.
3 = Tends to fall back and may have to try more than one time, but can get up without help.
4 = Unable to arise without help.

28. *Posture*
0 = Normal erect.
1 = Not quite erect, slightly stooped posture; could be normal for older person.
2 = Moderately stooped posture, definitely abnormal; can be slightly leaning to one side.
3 = Severely stooped posture with kyphosis; can be moderately leaning to one side.
4 = Marked flexion with extreme abnormality of posture.

29. *Gait*
0 = Normal.
1 = Walks slowly, may shuffle with short steps, but no festination (hastening steps) or propulsion.
2 = Walks with difficulty, but requires little or no assistance; may have some festination, short steps, or propulsion.
3 = Severe disturbance of gait, requiring assistance.
4 = Cannot walk at all, even with assistance.

30. *Postural stability* (response to sudden, strong posterior displacement produced by pull on shoulders while patient erect with eyes open and feet slightly apart. Patient is prepared.)
0 = Normal.
1 = Retropulsion, but recovers unaided.
2 = Absence of postural response; would fall if not caught by examiner.
3 = Very unstable, tends to lose balance spontaneously.
4 = Unable to stand without assistance.

31. *Body bradykinesia and hypokinesia* (combining slowness, hesitancy, decreased armswing, small amplitude, and poverty of movement in general.)
0 = None.
1 = Minimal slowness, giving movement a deliberate character; could be normal for some persons. Possibly reduced amplitude.
2 = Mild degree of slowness and poverty of movement which is definitely abnormal. Alternatively, some reduced amplitude.
3 = Moderate slowness, poverty or small amplitude of movement.
4 = Marked slowness, poverty or small amplitude of movement.

IV. Complications of Therapy (in the past week)
A. DYSKINESIAS
32. *Duration: What proportion of the waking day are dyskinesias present?* (Historical information.)
0 = None
1 = 1-25% of day.
2 = 26-50% of day.
3 = 51-75% of day.
4 = 76-100% of day.

33. Disability: How disabling are the dyskinesias? (Historical information; may be modified by office examination.)
0 = Not disabling.
1 = Mildly disabling.
2 = Moderately disabling.
3 = Severely disabling.
4 = Completely disabled.

34. Painful dyskinesias: how painful are the dyskinesias?
0 = No painful dyskinesias.
1 = Slight.
2 = Moderate.
3 = Severe.
4 = Marked.

35. Presence of early morning dystonia (Historical information.)
0 = No
1 = Yes

B. CLINICAL FLUCTUATIONS
36. Are "off" periods predictable?
0 = No
1 = Yes

37. Are "off" periods unpredictable?
0 = No
1 = Yes

38. Do "off" periods come on suddenly, within a few seconds?
0 = No
1 = Yes

39. What proportion of the waking day is the patient "off" on average?
0 = None
1 = 1-25% of day.
2 = 26-50% of day.
3 = 51-75% of day.
4 = 76-100% of day.

C. OTHER COMPLICATIONS
40. Does the patient have anorexia, nausea, or vomiting?
0 = No
1 = Yes

41. Any sleep disturbances, such as insomnia or hypersomnolence?
0 = No
1 = Yes

42. Does the patient have symptomatic orthostasis? (Record the patient's blood pressure, height and weight on the scoring form)
0 = No
1 = Yes

V. Modified Hoehn and Yahr staging

Stage 0 = No signs of disease.

Stage 1 = Unilateral disease.

Stage 1.5 = Unilateral plus axial involvement.

Stage 2 = Bilateral disease, without impairment of balance.

Stage 2.5 = Mild bilateral disease, with recovery on pull test.

Stage 3 = Mild to moderate bilateral disease; some postural instability; physically independent.

Stage 4 = Severe disability; still able to walk or stand unassisted.

Stage 5 = Wheelchair bound or bedridden unless aided.

VI. Schwab And England Activities Of Daily Living Scale

100% = Completely independent. Able to do all chores without slowness, difficulty or impairment. Essentially normal. Unaware of any difficulty.

90% = Completely independent. Able to do all chores with some degree of slowness, difficulty and impairment. Might take twice as long. Beginning to be aware of difficulty.

80% = Completely independent in most chores. Takes twice as long. Conscious of difficulty and slowness.

70% = Not completely independent. More difficulty with some chores. Three to four times as long in some. Must spend a large part of the day with chores.

60% = Some dependency. Can do most chores, but exceedingly slowly and with much effort. Errors; some impossible.

50% = More dependent. Help with half, slower, etc. Difficulty with everything.

40% = Very dependent. Can assist with all chores, but few alone.

30% = With effort, now and then does a few chores alone or begins alone. Much help needed.

20% = Nothing alone. Can be a slight help with some chores. Severe invalid.

10% = Totally dependent, helpless. Complete invalid.

0% = Vegetative functions such as swallowing, bladder and bowel functions are not functioning. Bedridden.

Reproduced with permission from Fahn et al [1]. (C) 1987 Macmillan Healthcare Information

References

1   Fahn S, Elton R, UPDRS program members. Unified Parkinson's disease rating scale. In: Fahn S, Marsden C, Goldstein M, Calne D, eds. *Recent developments in Parkinson's disease*. Florham Park, NJ: Macmillan Healthcare Information; 1987:153-163.

2   Movement Disorder Society Task Force on Rating Scales for Parkinson's Disease. The Unified Parkinson's Disease Rating Scale (UPDRS): status and recommendations. *Mov Disord*. 2003;18:738-750.

3   Martínez-Martín P, Benito-León J, Alonso F, et al. Patients', doctors', and caregivers' assessment of disability using the UPDRS-ADL section: are these ratings interchangeable? *Mov Disord*. 2003;18:985-992.

4   Louis ED, Lynch T, Marder K, Fahn S. Reliability of patient completion of the historical section of the Unified Parkinson's Disease Rating Scale. *Mov Disord*. 1996;11:185-192.

5   Martinez-Martin P, Forjaz MJ. Metric attributes of the unified Parkinson's disease rating scale 3.0 battery: Part I, feasibility, scaling assumptions, reliability, and precision. *Mov Disord*. 2006;21:1182-1188.

6   Stebbins GT, Goetz CG. Factor structure of the Unified Parkinson's Disease Rating Scale: Motor Examination section. *Mov Disord*. 1998;13:633-636.

7   Kroonenberg PM, Oort FJ, Stebbins GT, et al. Motor function in Parkinson's disease and supranuclear palsy: simultaneous factor analysis of a clinical scale in several populations. *BMC Med Res Methodol*. 2006;6:26.

8   Steffen T, Seney M. Test-retest reliability and minimal detectable change on balance and ambulation tests, the 36-item short-form health survey, and the unified Parkinson disease rating scale in people with parkinsonism. *Phys Ther*. 2008;88:733-746.

9 Van Hilten JJ, Van der Zwan AD, Zwinderman AH, Roos RA. Rating impairment and disability in Parkinson's disease: evaluation of the Unified Parkinson's Disease Rating Scale. *Mov Disord*. 1994;9:84-88.

10 Siderowf A, McDermott M, Kieburtz K, et al. Test-retest reliability of the unified Parkinson's disease rating scale in patients with early Parkinson's disease: results from a multicenter clinical trial. *Mov Disord*. 2002;17:758-763.

11 Forjaz MJ, Martinez-Martin P. Metric attributes of the unified Parkinson's disease rating scale 3.0 battery: part II, construct and content validity. *Mov Disord*. 2006;21:1892-1898.

12 Bennett DA, Shannon KM, Beckett LA, et al. Metric properties of nurses' ratings of parkinsonian signs with a modified Unified Parkinson's Disease Rating Scale. *Neurology*. 1997;49:1580-1587.

13 Goetz CG, Stebbins GT, Chmura TA, et al. Teaching tape for the motor section of the unified Parkinson's disease rating scale. *Mov Disord*. 1995;10:263-266.

14 Kompoliti K, Comella CL, Goetz CG. Clinical rating scales in movement disorders. In: Jankovic J, Tolosa E, ed. *Parkinson's Disease and Movement Disorders*. Philadelphia, PA: Lippincott Williams and Wilkins; 2007: 692-701.

15 Goetz CG, Tilley BC, Shaftman SR, et al. Movement Disorder Society-sponsored revision of the Unified Parkinson's Disease Rating Scale (MDS-UPDRS): scale presentation and clinimetric testing results. *Mov Disord*. 2008;23:2129-2170.

16 Goetz CG, Fahn S, Martinez-Martin P, et al. Movement Disorder Society-sponsored revision of the Unified Parkinson's Disease Rating Scale (MDS-UPDRS): Process, format, and clinimetric testing plan. *Mov Disord*. 2007;22:41-47.

17 Martinez-Martin P, Alvarez-Sanchez M, Arakaki T, et al. Attributes related with the MDS-UPDRS Spanish version construct validity. *Mov Disord*. 2012;2(suppl 1):S100-S101.

18 Antonini A, Abbruzzese G, Ferini-Strambi L, et al. Validation of the Italian version of the Movement Disorder Society-Unified Parkinson's Disease Rating Scale. *Neurol Sci*. 2012;34(5):683-687.

19 Martinez-Martin P, Rodriguez-Blazquez C, Alvarez-Sanchez M, et al. Expanded and independent validation of the Movement Disorder Society-Unified Parkinson's Disease Rating Scale (MDS-UPDRS). *J Neurol*. 2013;260:228-236.

20 Gallagher DA, Goetz CG, Stebbins G, et al. Validation of the MDS-UPDRS Part I for nonmotor symptoms in Parkinson's disease. *Mov Disord*. 2012;27:79-83.

21 Martinez-Martin P, Ray Chaudhuri K, Rojo-Abuin JM, et al. Assessing the non-motor symptoms of Parkinson's disease: MDS-UPDRS and NMS Scale. *Eur J Neurol*. 2013. In press DOI: 10.1111/ene.12165 [Epub ahead of print].

22 McNeely ME, Duncan RP, Earhart GM. Medication improves balance and complex gait performance in Parkinson disease. *Gait Posture*. 2012;36:144-148.

23 Merello M, Gerschcovich ER, Ballesteros D, Cerquetti D. Correlation between the Movement Disorders Society Unified Parkinson's Disease rating scale (MDS-UPDRS) and the Unified Parkinson's Disease rating scale (UPDRS) during L-dopa acute challenge. *Parkinsonism Relat Disord*. 2011;17:705-707.

24 Schrader C, Capelle H-H, Kinfe TM, et al. GPi-DBS may induce a hypokinetic gait disorder with freezing of gait in patients with dystonia. *Neurology*. 2011;77:483-488.

25 Verbaan D, Van Rooden SM, Benit CP, et al. SPES/SCOPA and MDS-UPDRS: formulas for converting scores of two motor scales in Parkinson's disease. *Parkinsonism Relat Disord*. 2011;17:632-634.

26 Goetz CG, Stebbins GT, Tilley BC. Calibration of Unified Parkinson's Disease Rating Scale scores to Movement Disorder Society-Unified Parkinson's Disease Rating Scale scores. *Mov Disord*. 2012;27:1239-1242.

27 Goetz CG, Stebbins GT, LaPelle N, et al. MDS-UPDRS non-English translation program. *Mov Disord*. 2012;27(suppl 1):S96.

28 Goetz CG, Stebbins GT, Chmura TA, et al. Teaching program for the Movement Disorder Society-sponsored revision of the Unified Parkinson's Disease Rating Scale: (MDS-UPDRS). *Mov Disord*. 2010;25:1190-1194.

3. Global severity assessments

The Hoehn & Yahr Staging Scale (HY) represents the universally accepted system to classify patients based on their motor impairment and functional status. The Clinical Impression of Severity Index for Parkinson's Disease (CISI-PD) scale provides a clinical judgment on Parkinson's disease (PD) severity based on motor symptoms and complications, cognitive status, and disability.

Hoehn & Yahr Staging Scale (HY)	
Original, five-point version [1]	
Modified, seven-point version [2]	
Description of scale	
Overview	It assesses PD severity, with a focus on impairment (objective signs on examination) and disability (functional deficits)
	Formed by one single item, with five (original) or seven (modified) answer options. A short description is provided for each response option. The response options for the original version range from stages 1.0 to 5.0, and two half-step options were added in modified version: stages 1.5 and 2.5
	Completion time: about one minute, once the patient's functional and clinical states are known. Health professional-rated
	Time frame: time of assessment
	Specific for PD
Copyright?	Public domain
How can the scale be obtained?	The modified version can be found online, and in papers [3]
Clinimetric properties of scale in patients with PD	
Feasibility	Appropriate for PD population
	Applicable across all PD stages
Dimensionality	Not applicable
Acceptability	There is coincidence between possible and observed score ranges. Floor and ceiling effects are low for the modified version [4]
Reliability	The original HY has moderate inter-rater reliability [3]. No data available on test-retest reliability
Validity	Content validity: inadequate content validity for the HY as a whole, although all scale points except 2.5 were rated as having adequate content validity [5]
	Convergent validity with the Unified Parkinson's Disease Rating Scale (UPDRS) and Schwab & England Activities of Daily Living Scale (SE) was moderate/high. The HY also shows significant associations with measures of quality of life, objective motor performance, functional disability, and indices of dopaminergic activity [3,5,6]

© Springer Healthcare 2014

P. Martinez-Martin et al., *Guide to Assessment Scales in Parkinson's Disease*,
DOI: 10.1007/978-1-907673-88-7_3

Responsiveness & Interpretability	In a sample of 87 patients with PD followed for 2.6 years, 68% of patients increased at least 0.5 in HY stage [7]. It shows low sensitivity to change, especially in the lower stages [8]
	Valid for both sexes and all ages
Cross-cultural Adaptations & Others	Very widely used, and available in many languages
Overall impression	
Advantages	Simple and widely used by researchers and clinicians as the standard staging system; large body of research supporting the HY usefulness
Disadvantages	Dual focus on impairment and disability; it is weighted towards postural instability; low responsiveness, especially in early stages [3,8]

Clinical Impression of Severity Index for Parkinson's Disease (CISI-PD) (Figure 3.1) [9]	
Description of scale	
Overview	A severity index formed by four items (motor signs, disability, motor complications and cognitive status), rated 0 (not at all) to six (very severe or severely disabled). A total score is calculated by summing the item scores
	Time frame: time of assessment
	The scale is completed by a clinician. It takes a few seconds to complete [9] once the state of the patient is known
	Specific for PD
Copyright?	Public domain
How can the scale be obtained?	Available in the original publication [9]
Clinimetric properties of scale in patients with PD	
Feasibility	The CISI-PD items are appropriate for patients with PD. Applicable across all PD stages
Dimensionality	Unidimensional (by exploratory and confirmatory factor analyses) [9,10]
Acceptability	No floor or ceiling effect; satisfactory skewness [9,10]
Reliability	Internal consistency: satisfactory, with high Cronbach's alpha and item homogeneity [9,10]. Adequate test-retest reliability (intraclass correlation coefficient, ICC=0.84) [10]
Validity	Face/content validity is appropriate. Convergent validity with UPDRS, Scales for Outcomes in Parkinson's Disease-Motor (SCOPA-Motor), SCOPA-Cognition (SCOPA-Cog), SCOPA-Psychosocial (SCOPE-PS), Hospital Anxiety and Depression Scale (HADS), HY, SE, and CISI-PD was satisfactory [9,10]. The CISI-PD was used in clinimetric studies for many other PD scales [11–18]. The CISI-PD score is significantly influenced by disease duration, depression, HY stage, and disease duration [9,10]
Responsiveness & Interpretability	Not assessed. Valid for both sexes and all ages
Cross-cultural Adaptations & Others	Available in Spanish and English

Overall impression

Advantages	Simplicity and easy application; provides a global score, as well as a profile in specific components that are critical in PD
Disadvantages	Further studies should focus on attributes such as inter-rater reliability and responsiveness

---

Figure 3.1 Clinical Impression of Severity Index (CISI-PD)*

Motor Signs

0 Normal
1 Very mild
2 Mild
3 Mild to moderate
4 Moderate
5 Severe
6 Very severe

Disability

0 Normal
1 Minimal slowness and/ or clumsiness
2 Slowness and/ or clumsiness. No limitations
3 Limitation for demanding activities
   Does not need help, or rarely, for basic activities of daily living (ADL)
4 Limitation to perform basic ADL
   Help is required for some basic ADL
5 Great limitation to perform basic ADL
   Help is required for most or all basic ADL
6 Severely disabled; helpless
   Complete assistance needed

Motor Complications (dyskinesia and fluctuations)

0 Not at all
1 Very mild
2 Mild
3 Mild to moderate
4 Moderate
5 Severe
6 Very severe

Cognitive Status

0 Normal
1 Minimal cognitive problems
2 Mild cognitive problems. No limitations
3 Mild to moderate cognitive problems. Limitations for demanding activities. Does not need help, or rarely, for basic activities
4 Moderate cognitive problems. Limitations for basic activities. Help is needed for some basic activities
5 Severe cognitive problems. Many limitations for basic activities. Help is needed for most or all basic ADL
6 Severely disabled; helpless. Complete and continued assistance needed

---

	Score
Motor signs	_____
Disability	_____
Motor Complications	_____
Cognitive Status	_____

CISI-PD Total score (Sum of the four items (0-24)):

*Validation study published in *Mov Disord*. 2009;24:211-217. Scale reproduced with permission from Martinez-Martin et al [9]. ©2005 Movement Disorder Society

References

1 Hoehn MM, Yahr MD. Parkinsonism: Onset, progression and mortality. *Neurology*. 2001;57(suppl 3):S11-S26.

2 Fahn S, Elton R, UPDRS program members. Unified Parkinson's disease rating scale. In: Fahn S, Marsden C, Goldstein M, Calne D, eds. *Recent developments in Parkinson's disease*. Florham Park, NJ: Macmillan Healthcare Information; 1987: 153-163.

3 Goetz CG, Poewe W, Rascol O, et al. Movement Disorder Society Task Force report on the Hoehn and Yahr staging scale: status and recommendations. *Mov Disord*. 2004;19:1020-1028.

4 Martinez-Martin P, Forjaz MJ. Metric attributes of the unified Parkinson's disease rating scale 3.0 battery: Part I, feasibility, scaling assumptions, reliability, and precision. *Mov Disord*. 2006;21:1182-1188.

5 Forjaz MJ, Martinez-Martin P. Metric attributes of the unified Parkinson's disease rating scale 3.0 battery: part II, construct and content validity. *Mov Disord*. 2006;21:1892-1898.

6 Vingerhoets FJ, Snow BJ, Lee CS, et al. Longitudinal fluorodopa positron emission tomographic studies of the evolution of idiopathic parkinsonism. *Ann Neurol*. 1994;36:759-764.

7 Martinez-Martin P, Prieto L, Forjaz MJ. Longitudinal metric properties of disability rating scales for Parkinson's disease. *Value Health*. 2006;9:386-393.

8 Diamond SG, Markham CH. Evaluating the evaluations: or how to weigh the scales of parkinsonian disability. *Neurology*. 1983;33:1098-1099.

9 Martinez-Martin P, Forjaz MJ, Cubo E, et al. Global versus factor-related impression of severity in Parkinson's disease: a new clinimetric index (CISI-PD). *Mov Disord*. 2006;21:208-214.

10 Martínez-Martín P, Rodríguez-Blázquez C, Forjaz MJ, De Pedro J. The Clinical Impression of Severity Index for Parkinson's Disease: international validation study. *Mov Disord*. 2009;24:211-217.

11 Serrano-Dueñas M, Calero B, Serrano S, et al. Psychometric attributes of the rating scale for gait evaluation in Parkinson's disease. *Mov Disord*. 2010;25:2121-2127.

12 Virués-Ortega J, Rodríguez-Blázquez C, Micheli F, et al. Cross-cultural evaluation of the modified Parkinson Psychosis Rating Scale across disease stages. *Mov Disord*. 2010;25:1391-1398.

13 Martinez-Martin P, Rodriguez-Blazquez C, Abe K, et al. International study on the psychometric attributes of the non-motor symptoms scale in Parkinson disease. *Neurology*. 2009;73:1584-1591.

14 Martínez-Martín P, Carroza-García E, Frades-Payo B, et al. [Psychometric attributes of the Scales for Outcomes in Parkinson's Disease-Psychosocial (SCOPA-PS): validation in Spain and review]. *Rev Neurol*. 2009;49:1-7.

15 Martínez-Martín P, Frades-Payo B, Rodríguez-Blázquez C, et al. [Psychometric attributes of Scales for Outcomes in Parkinson's Disease-Cognition (SCOPA-Cog), Castilian language]. *Rev Neurol*. 2008;47:337-343.

16 Virués-Ortega J, Carod-Artal FJ, Serrano-Dueñas M, et al. Cross-cultural validation of the Scales for Outcomes in Parkinson's Disease-Psychosocial questionnaire (SCOPA-PS) in four Latin American countries. *Value Health*. 2009;12:385-391.

17 Carod-Artal FJ, Martínez-Martin P, Kummer W, Ribeiro L da S. Psychometric attributes of the SCOPA-COG Brazilian version. *Mov Disord*. 2008;23:81-87.

18 Martinez-Martin P, Cubo-Delgado E, Aguilar-Barbera M, et al. [A pilot study on a specific measure for sleep disorders in Parkinson's disease: SCOPA-Sleep]. *Rev Neurol*. 2006;43:577-583.

4. Motor impairment and disability scales

An increasing number of scales used to assess Parkinson's disease (PD) motor manifestations (tremor, rigidity, bradykinesia) and disability have been developed in the past years. However, some of them lack appropriate validation. In this chapter, the most widely used and tested scales to assess motor manifestations and disability are discussed.

Scales for Outcomes in Parkinson's Disease-Motor (SCOPA-Motor) [1]	
Description of scale	
Overview	Composed of 21 items grouped into 3 sections: Motor impairment (10 items); activities of daily living (ADL) (7 items); and motor complications (4 items). Items are scored in a 4-point scale: from 0 (normal) to 3 (severe)
	Mean time to complete the scale: 8.1 (SD=1.9) minutes [1]
	Time frame:time of assessment, except for items nine and ten
	Rated by a specialized rater
	Specific for patients with PD
Copyright?	Owned by SCOPA-Propark Study
How can the scale be obtained?	The scale is available free of charge with the permission of the authors in the original publication [1] and in the website: www.scopa-propark.eu
Clinimetric properties of scale in patients with PD	
Feasibility	The scale has been applied to patients with PD across all stages [2]
Dimensionality	Multidimensional
Acceptability	No floor or ceiling effects, except floor effect in complications [2,3]
	Skewness was acceptable [3]
Reliability	Cronbach's alpha >0.90 for all sections [1–3]. Item-total corrected correlation and item homogeneity were satisfactory as a whole [1–3]
	Inter-rater reliability: moderate to substantial [1]
	Test-retest: kappa coefficients >0.80 in motor impairment section items [1]
Validity	Face/content validity: not tested
	Convergent validity: correlations between Unified Parkinson's Disease Rating Scale (UPDRS) and SCOPA-Motor related sections was very high [1]. Also, correlations with Hoehn & Yahr Staging Scale (HY) and Clinical Impression of Severity Index for Parkinson's Disease (CISI-PD) [3]
	Known-groups: significant differences in SCOPA-Motor sections scores by HY [2,3] and Clinical Global Impression (CGI) severity levels [2]
	Internal validity: not tested
Responsiveness & Interpretability	Standard error of measurement (SEM): from 0.40 (dyskinesias) to 2.62 (motor impairment) [2,3]

© Springer Healthcare 2014
P. Martinez-Martin et al., *Guide to Assessment Scales in Parkinson's Disease*,
DOI: 10.1007/978-1-907673-88-7_4

Cross-cultural Adaptations & Others	English, Dutch, Spanish, and Brazilian translations (www.scopa-propark.eu). The scale has been used in USA and several Latin-American countries with satisfactory clinimetric results [3,4]
Overall impression	
Advantages	Shorter and quicker to administer than UPDRS and Movement Disorders Society sponsored revision of the Unified Parkinson's Disease Rating Scale (MDS-UPDRS), with suitable clinimetric properties
Disadvantages	Lack of data on test-retest reliability and responsiveness; some flaws in motor impairment section

Schwab & England Activities of Daily Living Scale (SE) [5]	
Description of scale	
Overview	Assesses patient's perceived disability through an 11-response options scale from 0% (bedridden with vegetative functions) to 100% (completely independent). A short description is provided for each step
	Time to complete the scale: a few minutes
	Time frame: time of assessment
	It may be rated by the clinician or the patient [6]
	Not specifically developed for but widely applied in PD [7]
Copyright?	Public domain
How can the scale be obtained?	It is available in several websites, such as: www.parkinsons.va.gov/resources/SE.asp
Clinimetric properties of scale in patients with PD	
Feasibility	Applicable across all PD stages
	Missing data: 7% in one study [8]
Dimensionality	Not applicable
Acceptability	Possible and observable score range coincide; floor and ceiling effects lower than 10%. Score distribution is mildly skewed towards negative values [8,9]
Reliability	No information available
Validity	Content validity: low for the global scale; satisfactory for all scale levels except the midpoint [10]. Convergent validity with HY, UPDRS, and Intermediate Scale for Assessment of Parkinson's Disease (ISAPD): moderate to high [10–12]
Responsiveness & Interpretability	The SE was sensitive to change in a two-year follow-up study [9]
	The minimally clinical important difference was estimated in six points [9]
	The SE is valid for all age groups and both sexes
Cross-cultural Adaptations & Others	Widely used and available in many languages. No studies about cross-cultural validity
Overall impression	
Advantages	Simple; widely used
Disadvantages	Lack of standardization of administration [6]; limited information about its reliability

Rating Scale for Gait Evaluation (RSGE-PD)	
23-item (Figure 4.1) [13] and 21-items [14] versions are available	
Description of scale	
Overview	Specifically developed to evaluate gait in patients with PD [13]
	The second version consists of 21 items, grouped into 4 sections: functional ability; long-term complications; socioeconomic; and examination. Items are rated 0 to 3, and a short description is provided for each step [14]
	Time to complete the scale: around 10 minutes
	Time frame: the week before, except for the examination section (current)
	Clinician-rated
	Specific for PD
Copyright?	Public domain
How can the scale be obtained?	It is published in the original paper [13] and Version 2.0 is included in a Spanish book on PD [15]
Clinimetric properties of scale in patients with PD	
Feasibility	Questions are appropriate for PD, and the scale is applicable to all PD stages
Dimensionality	Factor analysis of the first version showed four factors (mobility/gait, socioeconomic aspects, rigidity, and complications) [13]
Acceptability	The RSGE-PD Version 2.0 does not show floor or ceiling effects, and skewness and kurtosis were within standards [16]
Reliability	Cronbach's alpha for the first version total scale was high, with a satisfactory inter-rater agreement for all items except axial rigidity [13]. Internal consistency of the second version was also appropriate (both for the domains and the total scale) [16]
Validity	The convergent validity of the first version was high with disability measures, as well as HY stage, UPDRS, and timed tests [13]. The second version showed a moderate-to-high convergent validity with disease and levodopa treatment duration [16]
	Version 2.0 displayed satisfactory known-groups validity by HY stage [16]
Responsiveness & Interpretability	No information available on responsiveness or interpretability
	Valid for both sexes. It was tested in sample populations with age range between 38 and 83 years of age. [13,16]
Cross-cultural Adaptations & Others	The RSGE-PD was developed and applied in Spanish [13,16]. There is an English version published [13]
Overall impression	
Advantages	It shows sound clinimetric properties and offers a global gait assessment
Disadvantages	Limited use; Has been criticized for being prone to observer bias, similarly to other clinical scales with subjective component [17]

Abnormal Involuntary Movement Scale (AIMS) [18]	
Description of scale	
Overview	Assessment of the severity of abnormal movements in different parts of the body: face, mouth, limbs, and trunk [18]. Includes three global assessments: overall severity, disability, and patient's awareness of dyskinesias
	Ten items rated on a 5-point scale, from 0 to 4 (absent, minimal, mild, moderate, severe). Maximum score is 40
	Time to complete the scale: 15 minutes (estimated) [19]
	Clinician-rated. Specific instructions are provided
	Originally developed for rating tardive dyskinesia, it has been used for PD-related dyskinesia, but only partly validated in this population [19]
Copyright?	Public domain
How can the scale be obtained?	Available in many Internet sites (for example: http://depts.washington.edu/dbpeds/Screening Tools/AIMS.pdf)
Clinimetric properties of scale in patients with PD	
Feasibility	Not tested, although it has been widely used in patients with PD [19]. No evidence that AIMS is able to detect dyskinesia severity across PD stages [19]
Dimensionality	Its structure has not been formally tested
Acceptability	Not available [19]
Reliability	Internal consistency: not assessed
	Inter-rater and test-retest reliability: high in patients without PD [20,21]. In patients with PD, a modified version (excluding facial and global ratings items) reached a correlation between raters of 0.81 [22]. In another study, inter-rater reliability of the modified version was acceptable [23]
Validity	Face/content validity: not assessed
	Convergent validity: AIMS correlated weakly-to-moderately with Parkinson's Disease Questionnaire – 39 items (PDQ-39) domains [24]. ACorrelation between a modified version of AIMS and Parkinson Disease Dyskinesia Scale (PDYS-26) [22] and moderately-to-high with continuous ambulatory multi-channel accelerometry [23]. Modified AIMS scores increases in relation to ADL tasks [23]
	No other types of validity tested
Responsiveness & Interpretability	The AIMS has been used to ascertain changes in dyskinesias following treatment or surgery in several PD studies [25,26]. It seems to be responsive to changes [19]
Cross-cultural Adaptations & Others	Modified versions have been used in patients with PD [23,24] but have not been formally validated
Overall impression	
Advantages	Easy and quick to administer; widely used in clinical trials; sensitive to changes [19]
Disadvantages	Lack of validation studies in patients with PD; emphasizes ratings for facial-oral-lingual areas and less for movements in limbs and trunk

Rush Dyskinesia Rating Scale (RDRS) [27]	
Description of scale	
Overview	Objective assessment of dyskinesia during activities of daily living
	RDRS assesses the interference of dyskinesia during three standardized motor tasks: walking, drinking from a cup, and dressing. Each task is rated on a 5-point scale for severity of dyskinesia, from 0 (absent) to 4 (violent dyskinesia, incompatible with any normal motor task). Additionally, the type of dyskinesia and which one is most disabling is recorded
	Time to complete the scale: 5 minutes (estimated) [19]
	Time frame: time of assessment
	Rated by a health professional
	Specific for PD
Copyright?	Public domain
How can the scale be obtained?	Available from the original publication [27] and in the MDS website: www.movementdisorders.org/publications/rating_scales/
Clinimetric properties of scale in patients with PD	
Feasibility	Designed and validated for PD, RDRS has been widely used in this setting [19]
	Applicability across PD stages not formally tested
Dimensionality	Not tested, but it is intended to assess a unique construct (eg, disability caused by dyskinesia)
Acceptability	Not reported
Reliability	Internal consistency: not reported
	Inter-rater reliability: high for severity of dyskinesia, moderate-low for type and most disabling dyskinesia ratings. Intra-rater agreement was high [27]
Validity	Not tested
Responsiveness & Interpretability	Although used in clinical trials, its sensitivity and responsiveness have not been formally tested [19]. The scale seems to detect changes in dyskinesia due to treatment [28]
Cross-cultural Adaptations & Others	Not reported
	Derived from the Obeso Dyskinesia Scale [29]
Overall impression	
Advantages	Short and easy to administer; assesses functional disability in a standardized way
Disadvantages	Lack of full formal validation; does not include pain/discomfort due to dyskinesia or patient's perceptions

The Wearing-Off Questionnaires (WOQ)
Several versions: Patient Questionnaire (WOQ-32) [30]; Patient Card Questionnaire (WOQ-19), known as the 'QUICK Questionnaire' (Spanish version) [31]; 9-item symptom questionnaire (WOQ-9) [32]; and a 10-item questionnaire (Q10) [33]

Description of scale

Overview	The WOQ questionnaires were developed as screening tools to identify patients with wearing-off. The number of items is specified in the name of the scales, with 9, 10, 19, or 32 items. There is also an 18-item version (WOQ-18), similar to the WOQ-19 but without the item 'Aching' [34]. The WOQ-19 and Q10 have six items in common, the former with a higher detection power for non-motor symptoms [33]. For each item, patients are asked to mark if they experience the symptom, and if it improves after the next medication dose. A positive response is considered when a symptom is reported to improve
	Time to complete the scale: around 5 (shorter version) to 15 minutes (longer versions), 6 to 7 minutes for the WOQ-10 [33]
	Time frame: time of assessment
	The questionnaires are completed by the patient
	Specifically developed and validated for PD
Copyright?	Public domain
How can the scale be obtained?	The WOQ-32 is published as an appendix to the original study [30]. The Spanish, Flemish, and Italian versions of the WOQ-19 have also been published [34–36]

Clinimetric properties of scale in patients with PD

Feasibility	The WOQ-18 and WOQ-19 were judged by clinicians as useful for detecting wearing-off symptoms [34,37]. The WOQ scales are applicable to all PD stages
Dimensionality	Not assessed
Acceptability	No information
Reliability	The internal consistency of the WOQ-19 was adequate and test-retest reliability was also appropriate [36]
Validity	Content validity is estimated to be adequate
	The WOQ-32 significantly differentiated between groups by duration of levodopa treatment [30], and the WOQ-19 by HY stage and education level [35]. The WOQ-19 total number of symptoms correlates moderately with quality of life [38]. Criterion validity was established for the WOQ-19, when compared to clinical diagnosis of wearing-off established by a neurologist [36]. The WOQ-32 and WOQ-19 identified more patients with wearing off than other methods [30,35]. The prevalence of symptoms assessed by the WOQ-10 increases significantly with increasing wearing-off severity rated by neurologists [33]
Responsiveness & Interpretability	The WOQ scales were used in some clinical trials as screening measures to identify wearing-off patients [38,39]. Both motor and non-motor symptoms, as identified by the WOQ-9, were sensitive to dopaminergic treatment [40]
	WOQ scales are valid for both sexes and all ages

Cross-cultural Adaptations & Others	Besides English [30] and Spanish [33,41], the WOQ has been translated and used in many languages such as French [42], Russian [39], Flemish [34], Chinese [43], Japanese [44], Italian [36], German [38], and Czech [45], among others [46]
Overall impression	
Advantages	Specific screening instruments for wearing-off, with adequate screening properties [47]; simplicity, ease, and short time of completion; very useful for clinical practice and research. WOQ-19 and WOQ-9 are "recommended" by the MDS-Task force for screening of wearing-off in PD [47]
Disadvantages	WOQ-32 was not intended for use in clinical practice and may cause patient fatigue in completing it [46]; WOQ 10 requires additional studies
	Some studies differ to each other in requiring one or two positive responses to diagnose wearing-off [33,46]

Figure 4.1 Rating Scale for Gait Evaluation in Parkinson's Disease (RSGE)

I **Functional ability (Historical; determine for "On/Off")**

1 Space where walking takes place
   0 Normal; the patient walks freely inside and outside the house
   1 The patient walks freely but with caution or accompanied outside the house, with few or no limitations
   2 Some help or support is needed inside the house. Activity outside is scarce or nil
   3 Incapacity or significant difficulty in walking inside, even when aided

2 Independence related to gait
   0 Normal
   1 Only the most demanding activites (walking quickly or with long steps, jumping some obstacles) are limited
   2 Some help is needed or there are limitations in performing activities that require movement (going for a walk, getting on a bus, passing from one room to another)
   3 Disabled; needs assistance to move

---

3 Arising from chair/getting out of bed
   0 Normal
   1 Mild slowing and /or difficulty but completely independent
   2 Moderate slowing and/or difficulty, can need support or some assistance to get up
   3 Unable to arise without help

4 Climbing stairs
   0 Normal
   1 Mild impairment but could be normal for an older person
   2 Moderately impaired (slowing, difficulty, fatiguing); occasionally may need assistance
   3 Needs significant assistance or cannot climb stairs at all

5 Walking
   0 Normal
   1 Mild slowing and/or difficulty
   2 Moderate slowing and/or difficulty, but requires little or no assistance
   3 Severe slowing and/or difficulty, requiring significant assistance or cannot walk even assisted

6 Falling
0 None
1 Rare falling
2 Occasionally falls, but less than once per day
3 Falls once per day or more

II Long-tern complications (Historical; in the past week)

7 Freezing episodes when walking
0 None
1 Occasional freezing, but there are no falls due to freezing
2 Frequent freezing; occasional falls due to freezing
3 Constantly present, giving rise to frequent falls or prevention of walking

8 "Off" episondes impairing gait
0 None
1 "Offs" impairing gait ≤1 h per day
2 "Offs" impairing gait 1–3 h in a day
3 "Offs" impairing gait >3 h in a day

9 Dyskinesias impairing gait
0 None
1 Mildly disabling
2 Moderately disabling (causing insecurity, lack of balance, accidents)
3 Severely disabling; can prevent walking

III Socioeconomic (Historical)

10 Activities of work or self-care
0 Normal
1 Mild slowing or difficulty in performance
2 Moderately impaired; some of these activities are no longer possible
3 Incapable of performing these activities

11 Economy (economic consequences of the disability due to the gait impairment)
0 Normal
1 Mildly affected as a consequence of limitations in job, public transport, shopping
2 Moderately affected by working troubles and/or costs of treatment, special transport, caregiver, structural adaptions at home
3 Significant economic consequences; social resources and institutional assistance may be needed

12 Leisure and social activites
0 Normal
1 Feasible only with mild difficulty
2 Only some activities are possible
3 Incapable of performing these activites

13 Family organization (effects of the disorder on the family organization and activities)
0 Normal
1 Mildly affected; minimal consequences or limitations
2 Moderately affected; the functional limitation of the patient have an influence on the family organization and activities
3 Severely affected; caring for the patient is the pivotal activity

IV Examination (at the time of visit)

14 Initiation (patient is instructed to initiate the gait, from standing, immediately after the order)
   0   Normal
   1   Mild slowing
   2   Moderate slowing; may have start hesitation
   3   Unable or severly impaired in initiating the gait

15 Festination
   0   None
   1   Occosional festination
   2   Frequent festination; occasional falls from festination
   3   Unable to walk or frequent falls from festination

16 Arm swing
   0   Normal
   1   Decreased arm swing (uni- or bilateral)
   2   Absence of arm swing (uni- or bilateral), but the upper extremities keep a normal posture
   3   Absence of arm swhing with flexion of upper extremites

17 Turns (180°)
   0   Normal
   1   Mild slowing or cautiousness; performed in one or two phases
   2   Moderate slowing or difficulty; performed in three or more phases
   3   Turns are very slowed and difficult or assistance is required

18 Balance while walking
   0   Normal
   1   Occasional impairment with self-adjustment or minimal support
   2   Moderately impaired; requires support (eg, stick) or mild assistance to walk; occasional falls due to imbalance.
   3   Severely impaired or unable to walk even when assisted; frequent falls due to imbalance

19 Arising from chair (patient attempts to arise from a straight-backed, 45 cm high, wood or metal chair with the wrists, semipronated, resting on the proximal thighs in a natural posture)
   0   Normal
   1   Mild slowing but sits upright at first attempt
   2   Needs more than one attempt and/or support (eg, from arms of seat) but needs assistance
   3   Unable to arise without help

20 Postural stability (response to sudden posterior displacement produced by pull on shoulders from behind while the patient is erect with eyes open and feet slightly apart [up to 30 cm]; patient is prepared)
   0   Normal
   1   Retropulsion, but recovers unaided
   2   Retropulsion without recovering; would fall if not caught by examiner
   3   Very unstable, tends to fall spontaneously or unable to stand without assistance

21   Rigidity in lower limbs (patient seated, relaxed, with feet side by side and with hips and knees flexed around 90°. The resistance to the passive abduction-adduction produced by means of the hands of examiner placed on the knees of patient is evaluated. It is recommended that this maneuver be performed with the examiner located at the side of, not facing, the patient)
      0   Absent
      1   Slight or barely detectable
      2   Moderate, but full range of motion is easily achieved
      3   Severe; range of motion is achieved with difficulty

22   Axial rigidity (resistance to the passive mobility of the neck is assessed)
      0   Absent
      1   Slight or barely detectable
      2   Moderate, but full range of motion is easily achieved
      3   Severe; range of motion is achieved with difficulty

23   Posture
      0   Normal
      1   Not quite erect, slightly stooped posture; it could be normal for an older person
      2   Moderately stooped posture, definitely abnormal; can be slightly leaning to one side
      3   Severely stooped posture; can be moderately leaning to one side

Reproduced with permission from: Martinez-Martin et al [13]. ©1997 Lippincott Williams and Wilkins

References

1   Marinus J, Visser M, Stiggelbout AM, et al. A short scale for the assessment of motor impairments and disabilities in Parkinson's disease: the SPES/SCOPA. *J Neurol Neurosurg Psychiatr*. 2004;75:388-395.
2   Martínez-Martín P, Benito-León J, Burguera JA, et al. The SCOPA-Motor Scale for assessment of Parkinson's disease is a consistent and valid measure. *J Clin Epidemiol*. 2005;58:674-679.
3   Forjaz MJ, Carod FJ, Virues J, et al. The SCOPA motor scale in Latin-America: Metric properties. *Mov Disord*. 2007;22:S193.
4   Wilson RE, Seeberger LC, Buck PO, et al. Investigation of the psychometric properties of the short Parkinson's evaluation scale/scales for outcomes in Parkinson's disease (SPES/SCOPA). *Mov Disord*. 2010;25:S348.
5   Schwab JF England AC. Projection technique for evaluating surgery in Parkinson's disease. In: Gillingham FJ, Donaldson MC, eds. *Third Symposium on Parkinson's Disease*. Edinburgh, Scotland: E & S Livingston. 1969;152-157
6   McRae C, Diem G, Vo A, et al. Schwab & England: Standardization of administration. *Mov Disord*. 2000;15:335-336.
7   Ramaker C, Marinus J, Stiggelbout AM, Van Hilten BJ. Systematic evaluation of rating scales for impairment and disability in Parkinson's disease. *Mov Disord*. 2002;17:867-876.
8   Martinez-Martin P, Forjaz MJ. Metric attributes of the unified Parkinson's disease rating scale 3.0 battery: Part I, feasibility, scaling assumptions, reliability, and precision. *Mov Disord*. 2006;21:1182-1188.
9   Martinez-Martin P, Prieto L, Forjaz MJ. Longitudinal metric properties of disability rating scales for Parkinson's disease. *Value Health*. 2006;9:386-393.
10   Forjaz MJ, Martinez-Martin P. Metric attributes of the unified Parkinson's disease rating scale 3.0 battery: part II, construct and content validity. *Mov Disord*. 2006;21:1892-1898.
11   Stebbins GT, Goetz CG. Factor structure of the Unified Parkinson's Disease Rating Scale: Motor Examination section. *Mov Disord*. 1998;13:633-636.
12   Martínez-Martín P, Gil-Nagel A, Morlán Gracia L, et al. Intermediate scale for assessment of Parkinson's disease. Characteristics and structure. *Parkinsonism Relat Disord*. 1995;1:97-102.

13 Martínez-Martín P, García Urra D, del Ser Quijano T, et al. A new clinical tool for gait evaluation in Parkinson's disease. *Clin Neuropharmacol.* 1997;20:183-194.

14 Martínez-Martín P, Cubo E. Scales to measure parkinsonism. In: Koller W, Melamed E, eds. *Handbook of Clinical Neurology: Parkinson's Disease and Related Disorders, Part I.* Edinburgh:Elsevier; 2007:291-327.

15 Molina J, González de la Aleja J, Bermejo-Pareja F, Martínez-Martín P. Trastornos del movimiento. I. Enfermedad de Parkinson y parkinsonismos. In: Bermejo-Pareja F, Porta-Etessam J, Díaz-Guzman J, Martínez-Martín P, eds. *Más de cien escalas en Neurología.* Madrid: Aula Médica; 2008:183-224.

16 Serrano-Dueñas M, Calero B, Serrano S, et al. Psychometric attributes of the rating scale for gait evaluation in Parkinson's disease. *Mov Disord.* 2010;25:2121-2127.

17 O'Sullivan JD, Said CM, Dillon LC, et al. Gait analysis in patients with Parkinson's disease and motor fluctuations: influence of levodopa and comparison with other measures of motor function. *Mov Disord.* 1998;13:900-906.

18 Guy W. Abnormal Involuntary Movement Scale. ECDEU Assessment manual for psychopharmacology. Revised. Rockville, MD: National Institure of Mental Health, US Department of Health, Education and Welfare; 1976.

19 Colosimo C, Martínez-Martín P, Fabbrini G, et al. Task force report on scales to assess dyskinesia in Parkinson's disease: critique and recommendations. *Mov Disord.* 2010;25:1131-1142.

20 Whall AL, Engle V, Edwards A, et al. Development of a screening program for tardive dyskinesia: feasibility issues. *Nurs Res.* 1983;32:151-156.

21 Sweet RA, DeSensi EG, Zubenko GS. Reliability and applicability of movement disorder rating scales in the elderly. *J Neuropsychiatry Clin Neurosci.* 1993;5:56-60.

22 Katzenschlager R, Schrag A, Evans A, et al. Quantifying the impact of dyskinesias in PD: the PDYS-26: a patient-based outcome measure. *Neurology.* 2007;69:555-563.

23 Hoff JI, Van den Plas AA, Wagemans EA, Van Hilten JJ. Accelerometric assessment of levodopa-induced dyskinesias in Parkinson's disease. *Mov Disord.* 2001;16:58-61.

24 Chapuis S, Ouchchane L, Metz O, et al. Impact of the motor complications of Parkinson's disease on the quality of life. *Mov Disord.* 2005;20:224-230.

25 Goetz CG, Damier P, Hicking C, et al. Sarizotan as a treatment for dyskinesias in Parkinson's disease: a double-blind placebo-controlled trial. *Mov Disord.* 2007;22:179-186.

26 Martínez-Martín P, Valldeoriola F, Tolosa E, et al. Bilateral subthalamic nucleus stimulation and quality of life in advanced Parkinson's disease. *Mov Disord.* 2002;17:372-377.

27 Goetz CG, Stebbins GT, Shale HM, et al. Utility of an objective dyskinesia rating scale for Parkinson's disease: inter- and intrarater reliability assessment. *Mov Disord.* 1994;9:390-394.

28 Sawada H, Oeda T, Kuno S, et al. Amantadine for dyskinesias in Parkinson's disease: a randomized controlled trial. *PLoS ONE.* 2010;5:e15298.

29 Obeso JA, Grandas F, Vaamonde J, et al. Motor complications associated with chronic levodopa therapy in Parkinson's disease. *Neurology.* 1989;39(suppl 2):11-19.

30 Stacy M, Bowron A, Guttman M, et al. Identification of motor and nonmotor wearing-off in Parkinson's disease: Comparison of a patient questionnaire versus a clinician assessment. *Mov Disord.* 2005;20:726-733.

31 Stacy M, Hauser R. Development of a Patient Questionnaire to facilitate recognition of motor and non-motor wearing-off in Parkinson's disease. *J Neural Transm.* 2007;114:211-217.

32 Stacy MA, Murphy JM, Greeley DR, et al; for the COMPASS-I Study Investigators. The sensitivity and specificity of the 9-item Wearing-off Questionnaire. *Parkinsonism Relat Disord.* 2008;14:205-212.

33 Martinez-Martin P, Hernandez B. The Q10 questionnaire for detection of wearing-off phenomena in Parkinson's disease. *Parkinsonism Relat Disord.* 2012;18:382-385.

34 Santens P, De Noordhout AM. Detection of motor and non-motor symptoms of end-of dose wearing-off in Parkinson's disease using a dedicated questionnaire: a Belgian multicenter survey. *Acta Neurol Belg.* 2006;106:137-141.

35 Martínez-Martín P, Tolosa E, Hernández B, Badia X. The Patient Card questionnaire to identify wearing-off in Parkinson disease. *Clin Neuropharmacol.* 2007;30:266-275.

36 Abbruzzese G, Antonini A, Barone P, et al. Linguistic, psychometric validation and diagnostic ability assessment of an Italian version of a 19-item wearing-off questionnaire for wearing-off detection in Parkinson's disease. *Neurol Sci*. 2012;33:1319-1327.

37 Silburn PA, Mellick GD, Vieira BI, Danta G, Boyle RS, Herawati L. Utility of a patient survey in identifying fluctuations in early stage Parkinson's disease. *J Clin Neurosci*. 2008;15:1235-1239.

38 Eggert K, Skogar O, Amar K, et al. Direct switch from levodopa/benserazide or levodopa/carbidopa to levodopa/carbidopa/entacapone in Parkinson's disease patients with wearing-off: efficacy, safety and feasibility--an open-label, 6-week study. *J Neural Transm*. 2010;117:333-342.

39 Litvinenko IV, Odinak MM, Mogil'naia VI, Sologub OS, Sakharovskaia AA. [Direct switch from conventional levodopa to stalevo (levodopa/carbidopa/entacapone) improves quality of life in Parkinson's disease: results of an open-label clinical study]. *Zh Nevrol Psikhiatr Im S S Korsakova*. 2009;109:51-54.

40 Stacy MA, Murck H, Kroenke K. Responsiveness of motor and nonmotor symptoms of Parkinson disease to dopaminergic therapy. *Prog Neuropsychopharmacol Biol Psychiatry*. 2010;34:57-61.

41 Martinez-Martin P, Tolosa E, Hernandez B, Badia X; for the ValidQUICK Study Group. Validation of the "QUICK" questionnaire—A tool for diagnosis of "wearing-off" in patients with Parkinson's disease. *Mov Disord*. 2008;23:830-836.

42 Azulay JP, Durif F, Rogez R, Tranchant C, Bourdeix I, Rerat K. [Precoce survey: a new self-assessment patient card for early detection and management of Parkinson disease fluctuations]. *Rev Neurol (Paris)*. 2008;164:354-362.

43 Chan A, Cheung YF, Yeung MA, et al. A validation study of the Chinese wearing off questionnaire 9-symptom for Parkinson's disease. *Clin Neurol Neurosurg*. 2011;113:538-540.

44 Kondo T, Takahashi K. [Translation and linguistic validation of the Japanese version of the wearing-off questionnaires(WOQ-19 and WOQ-9)]. *Brain Nerve*. 2011;63:1285-1292.

45 Bareš M, Rektorová I, Jech R, et al. Does WOQ-9 help to recognize symptoms of non-motor wearing-off in Parkinson's disease? *J Neural Transm*. 2012;119:373-380.

46 Stacy M. The wearing-off phenomenon and the use of questionnaires to facilitate its recognition in Parkinson's disease. *J Neural Transm*. 2010;117:837-846.

47 Antonini A, Martinez-Martin P, Chaudhuri RK, et al. Wearing-off scales in Parkinson's disease: Critique and recommendations. *Mov Disord*. 2011;26:2169-2175.

5. Comprehensive non-motor symptoms assessments

There are two instruments available for assessing a wide variety of non-motor symptoms (NMS) that may be present in Parkinson's disease (PD). One is completed by the patient, and the other by the clinician. Once identified, some NMS may be assessed in more detail with specific scales, such as those described in Chapter 6.

Non-Motor Symptoms Questionnaire (NMS-Quest) (Figure 5.1) [1]	
Description of scale	
Overview	It is a screening questionnaire revealing the range of NMS in PD [2]
	The NMS-Quest is a self-completed questionnaire featuring responses as 'yes' and 'no' to each item. It is composed of 30 items grouped into 9 domains:
	I, Digestive (7 items);
	II, Urinary tract (2 items);
	III, Apathy/Attention/Memory (3 items); IV, Hallucinations/Delusions (2 items);
	V, Depression/Anxiety (2 items); VI, Sexual function (2 items);
	VII, Cardiovascular (2 items);
	VIII, Sleep disorders (5 items);
	IX, Miscellaneous (pain, weight change, swelling, seating, diplopia) (5 items) [2]
	Time frame: previous month
	Time for administration: 5-7 minutes
	The screening questionnaire is filled out by the patient/caregiver while waiting to be seen in the clinic. It is used specifically to identify NMS in PD
Copyright?	The Movement Disorder Society (MDS). (www.movementdisorders.org/publications/rating_scales/)
How can the scale be obtained?	The scale can be obtained from the original publication [2]
Clinimetric properties of scale in patients with PD	
Feasibility	Specifically designed for patients with PD
	Used in all stages of PD to identify whether the patient has any NMS [1]
	Vocabulary avoiding medical jargon and adapted to a seventh-grade level
	Designed to be applicable to patients with PD across various levels of disabilities [1,2]
	Scores (number of declared NMS) significantly increase with disease duration and Hoehn & Yahr Staging Scale (HY) [1]
Dimensionality	NMS-Quest has nine domains [2]

© Springer Healthcare 2014

P. Martinez-Martin et al., *Guide to Assessment Scales in Parkinson's Disease*, DOI: 10.1007/978-1-907673-88-7_5

Acceptability	An almost complete range of scores (0 to 28) with mean values around 10 were observed [1,2]
Reliability	Test-retest and inter-rater: not tested
Validity	Convergent: NMS-Quest score was highly correlated with NMSS (Non-Motor Symptoms Scale) total score and corresponding domains [3,4]. Correlationn of total NMS-Quest with HY stage was moderate ($r_s = 0.31$) and a lower correlation was found with disease duration (r_s <0.30) [1,2]
	Known-groups: total score significantly increased with increased age, disease duration, and severity of disease [1,2]
	Internal: interdomain correlation was poor to moderate (0.06 to 0.37) [2]
Responsiveness & Interpretability	Not tested
Cross-cultural Adaptations & Others	Translated and validated into many languages
Overall impression	
Advantages	Quick and easy screening tool, usable by the patient/caregiver to flag up NMS; 90% of patients and caregivers felt that the issues raised in the NMS-Quest were relevant to day-to-day life [1]
Disadvantages	It does not assess severity of symptoms or effect of treatment

Non-Motor Symptoms Scale (NMSS) [4]	
Description of scale	
Overview	It is a tool to quantify a wide range of NMS, each one scored for severity and frequency by the physician [5]
	It is composed of 30 items grouped into 9 domains: I, Cardiovascular (2 items); II, Sleep/Fatigue (4 items); III, Mood/Apathy (6 items); IV, Perceptual problems/Hallucinations (3 items); V, Attention/Memory (3 items); VI, Gastrointestinal tract (3 items); VII, Urinary (3 items); VIII, Sexual function (2 items); and IX, Miscellaneous (4 items)
	Time frame: Correlationn month
	Time for administration: 5 to 10 minutes
	The NMSS is rated by health professionals and obtained through clinical interview. The score for each item is based on a multiple of severity (from 0 to 3) and frequency scores (from 1 to 4)
Copyright?	The MDS (www.movementdisorders.org/publications/rating_scales/)
How can the scale be obtained?	The scale can be obtained from the original publication [4]. [Note: the correct denomination of the domain III is 'Mood/Apathy'] [6]
Clinimetric properties of scale in patients with PD	
Feasibility	Specifically designed for patients with PD [4,6]
	Used in all stages of PD to identify the severity and frequency of a patient's NMS
	Designed to be applicable to patients with PD across various levels of disabilities [5]. Scores significantly increase with severity of disease based on HY stages, NMS-Quest, and health-related quality of life assessments [4,6]
Dimensionality	An exploratory factor analysis supported the nine domain structure, explaining 63% of the variance [4]

Acceptability	The overall floor and ceiling effect of the total NMSS score were lower than 1%. Skewness was 1.2. The domains showed variable floor effect [4,6]
Reliability	Cronbach's alpha coefficient ranged from 0.44 to 0.85 and item homogeneity from 0.16 to 0.54
	The multi-trait scaling reached a success, and probable success rate was higher than 95% for all domains, except the Miscellaneous domain (47% success rate), which contained wide ranging, unrelated questions from diplopia to weight change
	Most of item-total correlations were higher than the criterion 0.30 (0.10 to 0.73), the lowest values corresponding to the Miscellaneous domain [4,6]
	With the exception of Cardiovascular and Sexual domains?, test-retest was satisfactory (>0.70) in both validation studies [4,6]
Validity	NMSS total score reached a high correlation with Scales for Outcomes in Parkinson's Disease-Autonomic (SCOPA-AUT) (r_s =0.64), Parkinson's Disease Questionnaire-39 Items (PDQ-39) (r_s =0.70), and EQ-5D Index (r_s =0.57)
	Correlation with other measures (HY, SCOPA-Motor, SCOPA-Psychiatric complications [SCOPA-PC], SCOPA-Cognition [SCOPA-Cog], Clinical Impression of Severity Index [CISI-PD], PD Sleep Scale, and EQ-5D Visual Analogue Scale [VAS]) was moderate-to-high
	NMSS domains showed a tight association with other measures for similar constructs: sleep/fatigue with PDSS, perceptual problems/hallucinations with SCOPA-PC, and attention/memory with CISI-PD cognition
	There were weak correlations between the corresponding domains and other scales for mood and frontal function assessment [4]
	The correlation with domains of the NMS Questionnaire ranged from 0.44 to 0.74 [4]
Responsiveness & Interpretability	Standard error of measurement (SEM) for the NMSS has been determined and is considered satisfactory (<½ SD at baseline) [4,6]
	The scale has been found sensitive to changes induced by advanced therapies [7,8]
Cross-cultural Adaptations & Others	Translated and validated into many languages [5]
Overall impression	
Advantages	Assesses a wide range of NMS that may occur in patients with PD; evaluates NMS that are severe but relatively infrequent and those less severe but persistent; those symptoms that are simultaneously persistent and severe have more relevance in the final score
Disadvantages	Due to its composition, the Miscellaneous domain displays poor clinimetric attributes; there is limited information about the scale's interpretability and responsiveness

Figure 5.1 Non-Motor Symptoms Questionnaire (NMS-Quest)

Name	Date	Age
Centre ID	Male/Female	

Non-Movement Problems In Parkinson's

The movement symptoms of Parkinson's disease are well known. However, other problems can sometimes occur as part of the condition or its treatment. It is important that the doctor knows about these, particularly if they are troublesome for you.

A range of problems is listed below. Please tick the box 'Yes' if you have experienced it during the past month. The doctor or nurse may ask you some questions to help decide. If you have not experienced the problem in the past month, tick the 'No' box. You should answer 'No' even if you have had the problem in the past but not in the past month.

	Have you experienced any of the following in the last month?	Y	N
1	Dribbling of saliva during the daytime		
2	Loss or change in your ability to taste or smell		
3	Difficulty swallowing food or drink or problems with choking		
4	Vomiting or feelings of sickness (nausea)		
5	Constipation (less than 3 bowel movements a week) or having to strain to pass a stool (faeces)		
6	Bowel (fecal) incontinence		
7	Feeling that your bowel emptying is incomplete after having been to the toilet		
8	A sense of urgency to pass urine makes you rush to the toilet		
9	Getting up regularly at night to pass urine		
10	Unexplained pains (not due to known conditions such as arthritis)		
11	Unexplained change in weight (not due to change in diet)		
12	Problems remembering things that have happened recently or forgetting to do things		
13	Loss of interest in what is happening around you or doing things		
14	Seeing or hearing things that you know or are told are not there		
15	Difficulty concentrating or staying focussed		
16	Feeling sad, 'low' or 'blue'		
17	Feeling anxious, frightened or panicky		
18	Feeling less interested or more interested in sex		
19	Finding it difficult to have sex when you try		
20	Feeling light headed, dizzy or weak standing from sitting or lying		
21	Falling		
22	Finding it difficult to stay awake during activities such as working, driving or eating		
23	Difficulty getting to sleep at night or staying asleep at night		
24	Intense, vivid or frightening dreams		
25	Talking or moving about in your sleep as if you are 'acting' out a dream		
26	Unpleasant sensations in your legs at night or while resting, and a feeling that you need to move		
27	Swelling of your legs		
28	Excessive sweating		
29	Double vision		
30	Believing things are happening to you that other people say are not true		

Developed and validated by the International PD Non Motor Group
For information contact: susanne.tluk@uhl.nhs.uk or alison.forbes@uhl.nhs.uk

References

1 Chaudhuri KR, Martinez-Martin P, Schapira AHV, et al. International multicenter pilot study of the first comprehensive self-completed nonmotor symptoms questionnaire for Parkinson's disease: the NMSQuest study. *Mov Disord*. 2006;21:916-923.

2 Martinez-Martin P, Schapira AHV, Stocchi F, et al. Prevalence of nonmotor symptoms in Parkinson's disease in an international setting; study using nonmotor symptoms questionnaire in 545 patients. *Mov Disord*. 2007;22:1623-1629.

3 Cervantes-Arriaga A, Rodríguez-Violante M, Villar-Velarde A, López-Gómez M, Corona T. [Metric properties of clinimetric indexes for non-motor dysfunction of Parkinson's disease in Mexican population]. *Rev Invest Clin*. 2010;62:8-14.

4 Chaudhuri KR, Martinez-Martin P, Brown RG, et al. The metric properties of a novel non-motor symptoms scale for Parkinson's disease: Results from an international pilot study. *Mov Disord*. 2007;22:1901-1911.

5 Chaudhuri KR, Martinez-Martin P. Quantitation of non-motor symptoms in Parkinson's disease. *Eur J Neurol*. 2008;15(suppl 2):2-7.

6 Martinez-Martin P, Rodriguez-Blazquez C, Abe K, et al. International study on the psychometric attributes of the non-motor symptoms scale in Parkinson disease. *Neurology*. 2009;73:1584-1591.

7 Martinez-Martin P, Reddy P, Antonini A, et al. Chronic Subcutaneous Infusion Therapy with Apomorphine in advanced Parkinson's disease compared to conventional therapy: a real life study of non motor effect. *J Parkinsons Dis*. 2011;1:197-203.

8 Reddy P, Martinez-Martin P, Rizos A, et al. Intrajejunal levodopa versus conventional therapy in Parkinson disease: motor and nonmotor effects. *Clin Neuropharmacol*. 2012;35:205-207.

6. Scales that evaluate specific non-motor disorders

This chapter presents scales that evaluate two non-motor disorders frequently present in patients with Parkinson's disease (PD) : sleep problems and fatigue. In addition, a PD-specific scale that focuses on autonomic symptoms is reviewed.

Parkinson's Disease Sleep Scale (PDSS) [1] A revised version, the PDSS-2, has been developed (Figure 6.1) [2]. This review will consider mainly the original version, which has been more thoroughly tested and used	
Description of scale	
Overview	PDSS assesses nocturnal problems, sleep disturbances, and excessive daytime sleepiness
	It is composed of 15 items, addressing nocturnal symptoms commonly associated with PD (insomnia, nocturia, nocturnal motor symptoms, etc). Each item is rated on a visual analogue scale (VAS) from 0 (severe or always present) to 10 (never or not present). PDSS-2 is focused only on nocturnal sleep problems and items are scored from 0 (never) to 4 (very frequent). In both versions, total score is obtained by summing the items
	Time to complete the scale: a few minutes
	Time frame: the previous week
	Self-assessed
	Specific for PD
Copyright?	Public domain
How can the scale be obtained?	It can be obtained from the original publication [1]
Clinimetric properties of scale in patients with PD	
Feasibility	The scale includes some of the most common sleep disturbances in patients with PD based on the authors' experience [2]. Extensively used and validated in patients with PD in all severity stages [3]
Dimensionality	Factor analysis identified one factor accounting for 65% of the variance [4]. Confirmatory factor analysis has not been carried out
Acceptability	PDSS does not show floor or ceiling effects [1,4–6]. Patient responses do not cover the full range of scores [1,4,5]
Reliability	Internal consistency: PDSS Cronbach's alpha is high (>0.70 in most studies) [5–7], with an adequate item-total correlation and item homogeneity as a whole [4–7]
	Inter-rater reliability: not tested
	Test-retest reliability: satisfactory [1,4,6–8]

© Springer Healthcare 2014
P. Martinez-Martin et al., *Guide to Assessment Scales in Parkinson's Disease*,
DOI: 10.1007/978-1-907673-88-7_6

Validity	Face/content validity: not formally tested; by original authors stated that the 15 items chosen were based on an audit of their experiences in relation to sleep disturbances in over 800 patients with PD in addition to the reports of caregivers [1]
	Convergent validity: PDSS showed high correlations with Scales for Outcomes in Parkinson's Disease-Sleep (SCOPA-S) Nocturnal Sleep subscale [5], Pittsburgh Sleep Quality Index (PSQI), and (PDSS item 15) Epworth Sleepiness Scale (ESS) [1,6–9]. Total score correlated with sleep efficiency measured by polysomnography [9]. Moderate-to-high correlations with depression and health-related quality of life rating scales [4,6,8]
	Known-groups: significant differences in PDSS scores among patients grouped by Hoehn & Yahr Staging Scale (HY) severity levels and disease duration [5]. It discriminates between patients and controls [1,6] and between patients who do and do not experience sleep disturbances [1,6,9]
	Cutoff values for identifying patients with sleep problems have been calculated [5,9]
Responsiveness & Interpretability	Standard error of measurement (SEM) was 9.5 to 9.8 for cross-sectional data [4,5] and ranged from 1.8 to 5.01 for longitudinal data [4,6]
	Minimal important difference (MID) not calculated
	PDSS has demonstrated sensitivity to change in response to treatment [3,10]
Cross-cultural Adaptations & Others	Validated and translated into several languages [4,6,7,9]
Overall impression	
Advantages	Extensively used and validated; brief; responsive to changes; recommended by the Movement Disorders Society (MDS) Task Force [3]
Disadvantages	Does not include specific sleep disorders such as sleep apnea; the use of the VAS may require instruction [3]
	Most of these disadvantages have been overcome by the PDSS-2 [2]

Scales for Outcomes in Parkinson's Disease –Sleep (SCOPA-S) (Figure 6.2) [11]	
Description of scale	
Overview	It assesses nighttime sleep (NS) and daytime sleepiness (DS) in two subscales with response options ranging from 0 (not at all) to 3 (a lot). The NS subscale contains five items that address to sleep initiation, fragmentation, efficiency and duration, and early wakening. The maximum score is 15, with higher scores reflecting more severe sleep problems. The DS subscale includes six items that address falling asleep unexpectedly or in particular situations, difficulties staying awake, and whether falling asleep in the daytime was considered a problem. The maximum score is 18, with higher scores reflecting more severe sleepiness. SCOPA-S also includes a single question on sleep quality, scored on a seven-point scale (ranging from slept very well to slept very badly), which is used separately as a global measure of nocturnal sleep quality
	Time to complete the scale: a few minutes
	Time frame: the past month
	Self-assessed
	Specific for PD
Copyright?	Public domain

How can the scale be obtained?	It can be obtained from the original publication [11] or in the SCOPA-Propark website: www.scopa-propark.eu

Clinimetric properties of scale in patients with PD

Feasibility	Items were judged by experts and piloted among patients with PD to assess comprehensibility and clarity [11]. It is applicable to patients with PD in all stages of severity [5,11,12]
Dimensionality	Exploratory factor analysis has revealed one factor each for both subscales [5,11], although in one study, two factors were identified for DS subscale [12]
Acceptability	Patients' responses covered the full range of scores in NS and DS items, but not in the subscales' total scores [5,11,12]. Both subscales' items showed a floor effect, but total scores did not show floor or ceiling effects. Skewness was within the accepted limits [5,11,12]
Reliability	Internal consistency: high Cronbach's alpha coefficient for both subscales [5,11–13]. Item-total corrected correlation was satisfactory except for item six in DS subscale [12]
	Test-retest reliability: satisfactory for both subscales [11]
	Inter-rater: not tested
Validity	Face/content validity: items were selected from the literature and tested among patients with PD [11]. Formal testing has been carried out, with satisfactory results [13]
	Convergent: NS subscale was strongly correlated with PSQI and PDSS [5,11,13]. DS subscale correlated with ESS [11,13] and with PDSS item 15 [12]. Correlations with health-related quality of life scales were low-to-moderate [12]
	Known-groups: not significant differences in NS or DS scores by disease severity (HY staging) [5,11]. Both subscales discriminated between patients and controls [11]
	Predictive: cutoff score values of 3/4 [11] or 6/7 [5] were calculated for NS subscale to separate good from bad sleepers. For DS, cutoff value was 4/5 [11]
Responsiveness & Interpretability	SEM was calculated for both subscales, resulting in 1.4 for the NS and 1.5 for the DS subscale [5]
	Mininal important difference not determined
Cross-cultural Adaptations & Others	Translated and validated into Spanish [12] and Thai [13]

Overall impression

Advantages	Short and easy to apply; complete validation studies in different settings; recommended by the MDS Task Force [3]
Disadvantages	Lack of studies on responsiveness; does not include questions on specific sleep problems such as restless legs syndrome

Epworth Sleepiness Scale (ESS) [14]	
Description of scale	
Overview	The ESS measures the general level of DS in adults [14]. Subjects are asked to rate the likelihood that they will doze off in eight daily situations. The items are scored on a 4-points scale ranging from 0 (would never doze) to 3 (high chance of dozing). The total score is made up by summing the items, with a maximum of 24
	Time to complete the scale: a few minutes
	Time frame: recent times
	Self-assessed
	Not specific for PD. Validated in patients with PD [11,15]
Copyright?	Public domain
How can the scale be obtained?	It can be obtained from the original publication [14]
Clinimetric properties of scale in patients with PD	
Feasibility	Although generic, application in patients with PD resulted in good data quality, with a high percentage of fully computable data [15]
Dimensionality	Exploratory factor analysis has identified one [16] or two factors [11,15] However, Rasch analysis supported the unidimensionality of the scale [15]
Acceptability	Floor and ceiling effects were absent [15]. Score distribution was as follows: median, 10; inter-quartile range: 6–13 [15]
Reliability	Internal consistency: high Cronbach's alpha coefficient (0.84-0.86) [11,15] Item-total correlation coefficients ranged 0.46–0.71 [11,15]
	Test-retest: not tested
	Inter-rater: not tested
Validity	Face/content: not formally tested
	Convergent: strong relationship with SCOPA-S DS [11], Unified Parkinson's Disease Rating Scale (UPDRS) [17], and laboratory tests of somnolence [18]
	Known-groups: higher ESS scores are associated with higher HY staging and UPDRS scores [19]. ESS can discriminate between patients with PD and controls [19]
	Predictive: a value of ESS>7 indicates excessive daytime somnolence [20], although other studies use ESS>8 or ESS>10 for excessive somnolence [19,21]
Responsiveness & Interpretability	SEM and minimal important difference have not been calculated
	ESS has been widely used to assess change in response to treatment [3]
Cross-cultural Adaptations & Others	ESS is available in several languages and has been validated in different populations and settings [3]. A modified version for use in PD has been proposed [20]
Overall impression	
Advantages	Extensively used and validated; responsive to changes; scale recommended by the MDS-Task Force [3]
Disadvantages	It does not include some disturbances such as 'sleep-attacks'; self-assessment is a limitation in patients who are not aware of short naps; may need to be administered by proxy in patients with dementia

Scales for Outcomes in Parkinson's Disease-Autonomic (SCOPA-AUT) (Figure 6.3) [22]	
Description of scale	
Overview	For assessment of autonomic dysfunction in patients with PD
	Composed of 25 items, grouped into 6 subscales: Cardiovascular (3 items), Gastrointestinal (7), Urinary (6), Thermoregulatory (4), Pupillomotor (1), and Sexual (2)
	Items are scored from 0 (never) to 3 (often). Maximum possible score is 69
	Time to complete the scale: 10 minutes (estimated) [23]
	Time frame: past month
	Self-completed
	Specific for patients with PD
Copyright?	Owned by SCOPA-Propark Study
How can the scale be obtained?	Available free of charge with permission of the authors in the original publication [22] and in: www.scopa-propark.eu
Clinimetric properties of scale in patients with PD	
Feasibility	The SCOPA-AUT discriminates between control, mild, moderate, and severe PD groups [23]
Dimensionality	Factor analysis did not replicate the original structure [24]. Unidimensional by Rasch analysis [25]
Acceptability	Observed range did not cover the maximum possible range [24,26]
	Sexual function items have a high percentage of 'not applicable' responses and a marked floor effect [22,24,26]. Floor effect was also present in cardiovascular, thermoregulatory, and pupillomotor domains [24,26]
	Skewness in Sexual domain for women [26]
Reliability	Internal consistency: Cronbach's alpha from 0.56 (thermoregulatory) to 0.95 (sexual, women) [24,26]. Item-total corrected correlation and item homogeneity ranged from weak to satisfactory [24]
	Inter-rater agreement: 85% [27]
	Test-retest reliability: variable for items and satisfactory for the domains and total score [22,26]
Validity	Content validity: not formally tested [23]
	Convergent: moderate correlations with HY, SCOPA-Motor, and Clinical Impression of Severity Index for Parkinson's Disease (CISI-PD) [24,26,28], high with Non-Motor Symptoms Scale (NMSS), Parkinson's Disease Questionnaire–39 items (PDQ-39) [26] and SCOPA-Psychosocial (SCOPA-PS) [24]. Moderate-to-high with corresponding NMSS domains [26]. No correlation with electrophysiological autonomic measures [29], 123-I-MIBG (Iodine- 123-Metaiodobenzylguanidine) cardiac scintigraphy [30] or cognitive assessments [24,31]
	Known-groups: satisfactory for HY stages [22,24,26], age, and duration of disease [24]. Pupillomotor and sexual function showed no discrimination [26]
	Internal validity: variable [24]

Responsiveness & Interpretability	SEM has been determined [24]
	Differential item functioning (DIF) by sex in item 2 (sialorrhea) and DIF by age in item 13 (nocturia) [25]. Older patients or those with PD were more likely to choose the 'not applicable' option in Sexual domain [22,24,26,28]
Cross-cultural Adaptations & Others	Available in several languages (Dutch, Spanish, English, Portuguese)
Overall impression	
Advantages	Sound clinimetric properties: Rasch analysis proved that it can be used as a linear metric scale through conversion of raw scores [25]; recommended by the MDS-Task force [23,32]
Disadvantages	Weaknesses in the internal consistency of some subscales; lack of data on responsiveness; some important domains are not included [32]

Fatigue Severity Scale (FSS) [33]	
Description of scale	
Overview	The FSS measures fatigue severity in a range of medical and neurologic disorders
	The scale comprises 9 questions with answers on a 7-point Likert scale (1: strongly disagree; to 7: strongly agree). The total FSS score represents the mean score of each of the nine items, yielding a score range between 1 and 7. Higher scores indicate a higher level of fatigue
	Time frame: the previous week
	It takes up to 5 minutes to complete and is a self-administered questionnaire
	Generic, but used and validated in PD populations [34,35]
Copyright?	Copyrighted but freely available from its developers for research or clinical purposes. Commercial entities are charged for use of the FSS
How can the scale be obtained?	The scale can be obtained on the following link: www.mainedo.com/pdfs/FSS.pdf
Clinimetric properties of scale in patients with PD	
Feasibility	The scale is applicable to patients with PD in all severity stages [34] and it discriminates patients with PD from healthy controls
Dimensionality	Unidimensional [34,36]
Acceptability	Good data quality, with few missing item responses and a high percentage of fully computable data [36]. Floor- and ceiling-effect were absent [36]
Reliability	Internal consistency: excellent reliability (Cronbach's alpha: 0.94) [36]. Observed interitem correlations in PD range from 0.27 to 0.78
	Test-retest: no significant changes in FSS scores when no clinical change was expected [36]
	Inter-rater: not tested

Validity	Content: not tested in PD
	Convergent: moderate to strong correlations with other fatigue measures (Functional Assessment of Chronic Illness Therapy [FACIT-F], Nottingham Health Profile-Energy level subscale [NHP-EN], Piper Fatigue Scale [PFS], and a one-question fatigue rating) [34]. Low correlations between the FSS and quality of life (PDQ-39, Medical Outcomes Study-Short Form -36 [SF-36]) and depression measures (Hamilton Depression Rating Scale [HAM-D]) [34]
	Known-groups: FSS discriminates between fatigued and non-fatigued patients as per the NHP-EN [36]
Responsiveness & Interpretability	The FSS is responsive to change with time and treatment in PD [34]
	MID has not been assessed in PD
	DIF by age for two items, but not by sex [36]
Cross-cultural Adaptations & Others	It has been translated to and validated in various languages and shows sound clinimetric properties in non-PD disorders as well as PD
Overall impression	
Advantages	Brevity and ease of administration; scale is recommended by the MDS Task Force [34]
Disadvantages	Lack of definition of the underlying construct; additional studies on its clinimetric properties in PD are needed [34,35]

Multidimensional Fatigue Inventory (MFI) [37]	
Description of scale	
Overview	The MFI is a 20-item self-report instrument designed to measure fatigue, covering the following dimensions: General Fatigue, Physical Fatigue, Mental Fatigue, Reduced Motivation, and Reduced Activity. Each dimension contains four items, with two items formulated in a positive and two formulated in a negative direction, scored in a five-point scale. Scores range from 4 to 20 for subscales, with higher scores indicating greater fatigue severity
	Time frame: recent
	Time to complete the scale: about 5–10 minutes
	Generic, but suitable to patients with PD [34]
Copyright?	The scale can be used free of charge for academic use on the condition that the original publication is properly referenced
How can the scale be obtained?	It can be obtained from the original paper [37]
Clinimetric properties of scale in patients with PD	
Feasibility	The MFI has been used in several studies in patients with PD [34]
Dimensionality	The five-factor original structure has been replicated in some studies but not in others [34]. In PD, a four-factor structure has been identified [38], combining general fatigue and physical fatigue as one factor
Acceptability	Appropriate, with no floor or ceiling-effects in the total score [38]

Reliability	Internal consistency: high Cronbach's alpha coefficients, ranging from 0.74 to 0.92 [38]
	Test-retest: satisfactory, with intraclass correlation coefficient (ICC) ranging from 0.65 to 0.81 [38]. Not adequate for the mental fatigue dimension [38]
	Inter-rater: not tested in PD
Validity	Content: not tested in PD
	Convergent: MFI is strongly associated with other measures of fatigue (Daily Fatigue Impact Scale [D-FIS], Visual Analogue Scale for Fatigue [VAS-F]) [39], and with measures of physical activity [40]
	Known-groups: no data available in PD
	Internal: not tested
Responsiveness & Interpretability	MFI has been used in randomized controlled trials as an outcome measure of fatigue, with discordant results [41,42]
	Smallest detectable change (SDC) has been calculated [38]
	Normative values for general population are available [43]
Cross-cultural Adaptations & Others	The scale is available in 15 languages
Overall impression	
Advantages	Short scale with sound clinimetric properties; recommended by the MDS Task Force [34]
Disadvantages	The proposed factor structure has not been confirmed in PD; needs additional studies in PD population

Parkinson's Fatigue Scale (PFS) (Figure 6.4) [44]

Description of scale

Overview	The PFS is a 16-item patient-rated scale assessing physical aspects of fatigue in patients with PD and its impact on daily function. The item response options range from one ('strongly disagree') to five ('strongly agree'). There are three scoring options: a total PFS score by item score average; a binary scoring method with positive scores for each item generated by 'agree' and 'strongly agree' responses; and a total PFS score (range 16 to 80) based on the sum of items scores, which is most often used
	Time frame: the 2 weeks prior to assessment
	Time to complete the scale: not estimated, but it is a short scale
	Specific for patients with PD
Copyright?	Public domain
How can the scale be obtained?	It can be obtained free of charge from its developer for academic use

Clinimetric properties of scale in patients with PD

Feasibility	It has been specifically designed for patients with PD [44]. It discriminates between patients and healthy controls [44]
Dimensionality	Unidimensional, supported by confirmatory factor analysis [44]

Acceptability	Floor and ceiling effects were absent in the average total score, but a clear ceiling effect was detected in the dichotomized score [45]. Good data quality [44]. Scaling assumptions were supported by the distribution of scores [45]
Reliability	Internal consistency: high Cronbach's alpha coefficient and satisfactory item-total-corrected correlation [44–46]
	Test-retest: moderate to high for both average and binary scoring methods [44]
	Inter-rater: not tested
Validity	Content: not formally tested
	Convergent: strong correlations with other fatigue measures (FSS, Rhoten Fatigue Scale [RFS], and FACIT-F) [44–46]
	Internal: adequate [44]
	Predictive: cutoff scores are provided in the original publication [44]
Responsiveness & Interpretability	It is responsive to changes due to treatment [47,48]
	Precision and MID not calculated
Cross-cultural Adaptations & Others	Swedish and Brazilian versions have been validated [45,46]
Overall impression	
Advantages	Short and easy to administer; recommended by the MDS Task Force [34]
Disadvantages	Potential overlap with mood and cognitive status; lack of data on responsiveness and interpretability

---

Figure 6.1 Parkinson's Disease Sleep Scale (PDSS-2)

Please rate the severity of the following based on your experiences during the past week (7days). Please make a cross in the answer box

	Very often 6-7 times per week	Often 4-5 times per week	Sometimes 2-3 days per week	Occasionally 1 day per week	Never
1 Overall, did you sleep well during the last week?					
2 Did you have difficulty falling asleep each night?					
3 Did you have difficulty staying asleep?					
4 Did you have restlessness of legs or arms at nights causing disruption of sleep?					
5 Was your sleep disturbed due to an urge to move your legs or arms?					
6 Did you suffer from distressing dreams at night?					

7 Did you suffer from distressing hallucinations at night (seeing or hearing things that you are told do not exist)?					
8 Did you get up at night to pass urine?					
9 Did you feel uncomfortable at night because you were unable to turn around in bed or move due to immobility?					
10 Did you feel pain in your arms or legs which woke you up whilst sleeping at night?					
11 Did you have muscle cramps in your arms or legs which woke you up whilst sleeping at night?					
12 Did you wake early in the morning with painful posturing of arms and legs?					
13 On waking, did you experience tremor?					
14 Did you feel tired and sleepy after waking in the morning?					
15 Did you wake up at night due to snoring or difficulties with breathing?					

Figure 6.2 Scales for Outcomes in Parkinson's Disease-Autonomic (SCOPA-AUT)

By means of this questionnaire, we would like to find out to what extent in the past month you have had problems with various bodily functions, such as difficulty passing urine, or excessive sweating. Answer the questions by placing a cross in the box which best reflects your situation. If you wish to change an answer, fill in the 'wrong' box and place a cross in the correct one. If you have used medication in the past month in relation to one or more of the problems mentioned, then the question refers to how you were while taking this medication. You can note the use of medication on the last page.

1 In the past month, have you had difficulty swallowing or have you choked?
☐ never ☐ sometimes ☐ regularly ☐ often

2 In the past month, has saliva dribbled out of your mouth?
☐ never ☐ sometimes ☐ regularly ☐ often

3 In the past month, has food ever become stuck in your throat?
☐ never ☐ sometimes ☐ regularly ☐ often

4 In the past month, did you ever have the feeling during a meal that you were full very quickly?
☐ never ☐ sometimes ☐ regularly ☐ often

5 Constipation is a blockage of the bowel, a condition in which someone has a bowel movement twice a week or less.

In the past month, have you had problems with constipation?
☐ never ☐ sometimes ☐ regularly ☐ often

6 In the past month, did you have to strain hard to pass stools?
☐ never ☐ sometimes ☐ regularly ☐ often

7 In the past month, have you had involuntary loss of stools?
☐ never ☐ sometimes ☐ regularly ☐ often

Questions 8 to 13 deal with problems with passing urine. If you use a catheter you can indicate this by placing a cross in the box "use cathether".

8 In the past month, have you had difficulty retaining urine?
☐ never ☐ sometimes ☐ regularly ☐ often ☐ use catheter

9 In the past month, have you had involuntary loss of urine?
☐ never ☐ sometimes ☐ regularly ☐ often ☐ use catheter

10 In the past month, have you had the feeling that after passing urine your bladder was not completely empty?
☐ never ☐ sometimes ☐ regularly ☐ often ☐ use catheter

11 In the past month, has the stream of urine been weak?
☐ never ☐ sometimes ☐ regularly ☐ often ☐ use catheter

12 In the past month, have you had to pass urine again within 2 hours of the previous time?
☐ never ☐ sometimes ☐ regularly ☐ often ☐ use catheter

13 In the past month, have you had to pass urine at night?
☐ never ☐ sometimes ☐ regularly ☐ often ☐ use catheter

14 In the past month, when standing up have you had the feeling of either becoming lightheaded, or no longer being able to see properly, or no longer being able to think clearly?
☐ never ☐ sometimes ☐ regularly ☐ often

15 In the past month, did you become light-headed after standing for some time?
☐ never ☐ sometimes ☐ regularly ☐ often

16 Have you fainted in the past 6 months?
☐ never ☐ sometimes ☐ regularly ☐ often

17 In the past month, have you ever perspired excessively during the day?
☐ never ☐ sometimes ☐ regularly ☐ often

18 In the past month, have you ever perspired excessively during the night?
☐ never ☐ sometimes ☐ regularly ☐ often

19 In the past month, have your eyes ever been over-sensitive to bright light?
☐ never   ☐ sometimes   ☐ regularly   ☐ often

20 In the past month, how often have you had trouble tolerating cold?
☐ never   ☐ sometimes   ☐ regularly   ☐ often

21 In the past month, how often have you had trouble tolerating heat?
☐ never   ☐ sometimes   ☐ regularly   ☐ often

The following questions are about sexuality. Although we are aware that sexuality is a highly intimate subject, we would still like you to answer these questions. For the questions on sexual activity, consider every form of sexual contact with a partner or masturbation (self-gratification). An extra response option has been added to these questions. Here you can indicate that the situation described has not been applicable to you in the past month, for example because you have not been sexually active.
Questions 22 and 23 are intended specifically for men, 24 and 25 for women.
The following 3 questions are only for men

22 In the past month, have you been impotent (unable to have or maintain an erection)?
☐ never   ☐ sometimes   ☐ regularly   ☐ often   ☐ not applicable

23 In the past month, how often have you been unable to ejaculate?
☐ never   ☐ sometimes   ☐ regularly   ☐ often   ☐ not applicable

23a In the past month, have you taken medication for an erection disorder? (If so, which medication?)
☐ no   ☐ yes

Proceed with question 26

The following 2 questions are only for women

24 In the past month, was your vagina too dry during sexual activity?
☐ never   ☐ sometimes   ☐ regularly   ☐ often   ☐ not applicable

25 In the past month, have you had difficulty reaching an orgasm?
☐ never   ☐ sometimes   ☐ regularly   ☐ often   ☐ not applicable

The following questions are for everyone
The questions below are about the use of medication for which you may have or have not needed a doctor's prescription. If you use medication, also give the name of the substance.

26 In the past month, have you used medication for:

a. constipation?
☐ no   ☐ yes

b. urinary problems?
☐ no   ☐ yes

c. blood pressure?
☐ no   ☐ yes

d. other symptoms (not symptoms related to Parkinson's disease)
☐ no   ☐ yes

Figure 6.3 Scales for Outcomes in Parkinson's Disease-Sleep (SCOPA-S)

By means of this questionnaire, we would like to find out to what extent *in the past month* you have had problems with sleeping. Some of the questions are about problems with sleeping *at night*, such as, for example, not being able to fall asleep or not managing to sleep on. Another set of questions is about problems with sleeping *during the day*, such as dozing off (too) easily and having trouble staying awake.

A. Use of sleeping tablets

A1. How often did you use sleeping tablets in the last months?
(prescribed by a physician or not)
☐ not at all   ☐ less than once a week   ☐ once or twice a week   ☐ more than 3 times a week

A2. Which sleeping tablets did you use in the last month?
name: _____   amount per month: _____   dose per tablet: _____
name: _____   amount per month: _____   dose per tablet: _____
name: _____   amount per month: _____   dose per tablet: _____

B. Sleeping at night
The questions below are for everyone and concern sleeping at night. If you have been using sleeping tablets, then the answer should reflect how you have slept while taking these tablets.

B1. In the past month, have you had trouble falling asleep when you went to bed at night?
☐ not at all   ☐ a little   ☐ quite a bit   ☐ a lot

B2. In the past month, to what extent do you feel that you have woken too often?
☐ not at all   ☐ a little   ☐ quite a bit   ☐ a lot

B3. In the past month, to what extent do you feel that you have been lying awake for too long at night?
☐ not at all   ☐ a little   ☐ quite a bit   ☐ a lot

B4. In the past month, to what extent do you feel that you have woken up too early in the morning?
☐ not at all   ☐ a little   ☐ quite a bit   ☐ a lot

B5. In the past month, to what extent do you feel you have had too little sleep at night?
☐ not at all   ☐ a little   ☐ quite a bit   ☐ a lot

C1. Overall, how well have you slept at night during the past month?
☐ very well ☐ well ☐ rather well ☐ not well but not badly ☐ rather badly ☐ badly ☐ very badly

D. Sleeping during the day and the evening

D1. How often in the past month have you fallen asleep unexpectedly either during the day or in the evening?

☐ never   ☐ sometimes   ☐ regularly   ☐ often

D2. How often in the past month have you fallen asleep while sitting peacefully?

☐ never   ☐ sometimes   ☐ regularly   ☐ often

D3. How often in the past month have you fallen asleep while watching TV or reading?

☐ never   ☐ sometimes   ☐ regularly   ☐ often

D4. How often in the past month have you fallen asleep while talking to someone?

☐ never   ☐ sometimes   ☐ regularly   ☐ often

D5. In the past month, have you had trouble staying awake during the day or in the evening?

☐ never   ☐ sometimes   ☐ regularly   ☐ often

D6. In the past month, have you experienced falling asleep during the day as a problem?

☐ never   ☐ sometimes   ☐ regularly   ☐ often

Permission for the reuse of this questionnaire was granted by Dr J. Marinus, from the original publication: Marinus J, Visser M, van Hilten JJ, Lammers GJ, Stiggelbout AM. Assessment of sleep and sleepiness in Parkinson disease. SLEEP 2003;26:1049-1054. ©2013 Associated Professional Sleep Societies, LLC.

Figure 6.4 Parkinson's Fatigue Scale (PFS)

Name _____ **Date** _____ **Sex** _____

1 = strongly disagree

2 = disagree

3 = do not agree or disagree

4 = agree

5 = strongly agree

Item	Response rating (1 to 5)
1 I have to rest during the day	
2 My life is restricted by fatigue	
3 I get tired more quickly than other people I know	
4 Fatigue is one of my three worst symptoms	
5 I feel completely exhausted	
6 Fatigue makes me reluctant to socialize	

7 Because of fatigue it takes me longer to get things done	
8 I have a feeling of 'heaviness'	
9 If I wasn't so tired I could do more things	
10 Everything I do is an effort	
11 I lack energy for much of the time	
12 I feel totally drained	
13 Fatigue makes it difficult for me to cope with everyday activities	
14 I feel tired even when I haven't done anything	
15 Because of fatigue I do less in my days than I would like	
16 I get so tired I want to lie down wherever I am	
Total score	

Reproduced with permission from: Brown et al [44]. ©2004, Elsevier, Ltd

References

1   Chaudhuri KR, Pal S, DiMarco A, et al. The Parkinson's disease sleep scale: a new instrument for assessing sleep and nocturnal disability in Parkinson's disease. *J Neurol Neurosurg Psychiatry*. 2002;73:629-635.

2   Trenkwalder C, Kohnen R, Högl B, et al. Parkinson's disease sleep scale—validation of the revised version PDSS-2. *Mov Disord*. 2011;26:644-652.

3   Högl B, Arnulf I, Comella C, et al. Scales to assess sleep impairment in Parkinson's disease: critique and recommendations. *Mov Disord*. 2010;2516:2704-2716.

4   Martínez-Martín P, Salvador C, Menéndez-Guisasola L, et al. Parkinson's Disease Sleep Scale: validation study of a Spanish version. *Mov Disord*. 2004;19:1226-1232.

5   Martinez-Martin P, Visser M, Rodriguez-Blazquez C, et al. SCOPA-sleep and PDSS: two scales for assessment of sleep disorder in Parkinson's disease. *Mov Disord*. 2008;23:1681-1688.

6   Pellecchia MT, Antonini A, Bonuccelli U, et al. Observational study of sleep-related disorders in Italian patients with Parkinson's disease: usefulness of the Italian version of Parkinson's disease sleep scale. *Neurol Sci* 2012;33:689-694.

7   Wang G, Cheng Q, Zeng J, et al. Sleep disorders in Chinese patients with Parkinson's disease: validation study of a Chinese version of Parkinson's disease sleep scale. *J Neurol Sci*. 2008;271:153-157.

8   Margis R, Donis K, Schönwald SV, et al. Psychometric properties of the Parkinson's Disease Sleep Scale—Brazilian version. *Parkinsonism Relat Disord*. 2009;15:495-499.

9   Uemura Y, Nomura T, Inoue Y, Yamawaki M, Yasui K, Nakashima K. Validation of the Parkinson's disease sleep scale in Japanese patients: a comparison study using the Pittsburgh Sleep Quality Index, the Epworth Sleepiness Scale and Polysomnography. *J Neurol Sci*. 2009;287:36-40.

10 Ray Chaudhuri K, Martinez-Martin P, Rolfe KA, et al. Improvements in nocturnal symptoms with ropinirole prolonged release in patients with advanced Parkinson's disease. *Eur J Neurol*. 2012;19:105-113.

11 Marinus J, Visser M, van Hilten JJ, Lammers GJ, Stiggelbout AM. Assessment of sleep and sleepiness in Parkinson disease. *Sleep*. 2003;26:1049-1054.

12 Martínez-Martín P, Cubo-Delgado E, Aguilar-Barberà M, et al. [A pilot study on a specific measure for sleep disorders in Parkinson's disease: SCOPA-Sleep]. *Rev Neurol.* 2006;43:577-583.

13 Setthawatcharawanich S, Limapichat K, Sathirapanya P, Phabphal K. Validation of the Thai SCOPA-sleep scale for assessment of sleep and sleepiness in patients with Parkinson's disease. *J Med Assoc Thai.* 2011;94:179-184.

14 Johns MW. A new method for measuring daytime sleepiness: the Epworth sleepiness scale. *Sleep.* 1991;14:540-545.

15 Hagell P, Broman J-E. Measurement properties and hierarchical item structure of the Epworth Sleepiness Scale in Parkinson's disease. *J Sleep Res.* 2007;16:102-109.

16 Johns MW. Reliability and factor analysis of the Epworth Sleepiness Scale. *Sleep.* 1992;15:376-381.

17 Furumoto H. Excessive daytime somnolence in Japanese patients with Parkinson's disease. *Eur J Neurol.* 2004;11:535-540.

18 Stavitsky K, Saurman JL, McNamara P, Cronin-Golomb A. Sleep in Parkinson's disease: a comparison of actigraphy and subjective measures. *Parkinsonism Relat Disord.* 2010;16:280-283.

19 Kumar S, Bhatia M, Behari M. Excessive daytime sleepiness in Parkinson's disease as assessed by Epworth Sleepiness Scale (ESS). *Sleep Med.* 2003;4:339-342.

20 Hobson DE, Lang AE, Martin WR, et al. Excessive daytime sleepiness and sudden-onset sleep in Parkinson disease: a survey by the Canadian Movement Disorders Group. *JAMA* 2002;287:455-463.

21 Brodsky MA, Godbold J, Roth T, Olanow CW. Sleepiness in Parkinson's disease: a controlled study. *Mov Disord.* 2003;18:668-672.

22 Visser M, Marinus J, Stiggelbout AM, Van Hilten JJ. Assessment of autonomic dysfunction in Parkinson's disease: the SCOPA-AUT. *Mov Disord.* 2004;19:1306-1312.

23 Evatt ML, Chaudhuri KR, Chou KL, et al. Dysautonomia rating scales in Parkinson's disease: sialorrhea, dysphagia, and constipation—critique and recommendations by movement disorders task force on rating scales for Parkinson's disease. *Mov Disord.* 2009;24:635-646.

24 Rodriguez-Blazquez C, Forjaz MJ, Frades-Payo B, et al. Independent validation of the scales for outcomes in Parkinson's disease-autonomic (SCOPA-AUT). *Eur J Neurol.* 2010;17:194-201.

25 Forjaz MJ, Ayala A, Rodriguez-Blazquez C, et al. Assessing autonomic symptoms of Parkinson's disease with the SCOPA-AUT: a new perspective from Rasch analysis. *Eur J Neurol.* 2010;17:273-279.

26 Carod-Artal FJ, Ribeiro L da S, Kummer W, Martinez-Martin P. Psychometric properties of the SCOPA-AUT Brazilian Portuguese version. *Mov Disord.* 2010;25:205-212.

27 Cervantes-Arriaga A, Rodriguez-Violante M, Lopez-Gomez M, et al. NMSQuest, NMSS and SCOPA-AUT metric properties in Mexican Parkinson's disease population. *Mov Disord.* 2009;24:S381.

28 Verbaan D, Marinus J, Visser M, et al. Patient-reported autonomic symptoms in Parkinson disease. *Neurology.* 2007;69:333-341.

29 Papapetropoulos S, Argyriou AA, Chroni E. No correlation between the clinical severity of autonomic symptoms (SCOPA-AUT) and electrophysiological test abnormalities in advanced Parkinson's disease. *Mov Disord.* 2006;21:430-431.

30 Berganzo K, Tijero B, Somme JH, Llorens V, et al. SCOPA-AUT scale in different parkinsonisms and its correlation with (123) I-MIBG cardiac scintigraphy. *Parkinsonism Relat Disord.* 2012;18:45-48.

31 Idiaquez J, Benarroch EE, Rosales H, et al. Autonomic and cognitive dysfunction in Parkinson's disease. *Clin Auton Res.* 2007;17:93-98.

32 Pavy-Le Traon A, Amarenco G, Duerr S, et al. The Movement Disorders task force review of dysautonomia rating scales in Parkinson's disease with regard to symptoms of orthostatic hypotension. *Mov Disord.* 2011;26:1985-1992.

33 Krupp LB, LaRocca NG, Muir-Nash J, Steinberg AD. The fatigue severity scale. Application to patients with multiple sclerosis and systemic lupus erythematosus. *Arch Neurol.* 1989;46:1121-1123.

34 Friedman JH, Alves G, Hagell P, et al. Fatigue rating scales critique and recommendations by the Movement Disorders Society task force on rating scales for Parkinson's disease. *Mov Disord.* 2010;25:805-822.

35 Elbers RG, Rietberg MB, Van Wegen EEH, et al. Self-report fatigue questionnaires in multiple sclerosis, Parkinson's disease and stroke: a systematic review of measurement properties. *Qual Life Res*. 2012;21:925-944.

36 Hagell P, Höglund A, Reimer J, et al. Measuring fatigue in Parkinson's disease: a psychometric study of two brief generic fatigue questionnaires. *J Pain Symptom Manage*. 2006;32:420-432.

37 Smets EM, Garssen B, Bonke B, De Haes JC. The Multidimensional Fatigue Inventory (MFI) psychometric qualities of an instrument to assess fatigue. *J Psychosom Res*. 1995;39:315-325.

38 Elbers RG, Van Wegen EEH, Verhoef J, Kwakkel G. Reliability and structural validity of the Multidimensional Fatigue Inventory (MFI) in patients with idiopathic Parkinson's disease. *Parkinsonism Relat Disord*. 2012;18:532-536.

39 Martinez-Martin P, Catalan MJ, Benito-Leon J, et al. Impact of fatigue in Parkinson's disease: the Fatigue Impact Scale for Daily Use (D-FIS). *Qual Life Res*. 2006;15:597-606.

40 Elbers R, Van Wegen EEH, Rochester L, et al. Is impact of fatigue an independent factor associated with physical activity in patients with idiopathic Parkinson's disease? *Mov Disord*. 2009;24:1512-1518.

41 Lou J-S, Kearns G, Benice T, et al. Levodopa improves physical fatigue in Parkinson's disease: a double-blind, placebo-controlled, crossover study. *Mov Disord*. 2003;18:1108-1114.

42 Mendonça DA, Menezes K, Jog MS. Methylphenidate improves fatigue scores in Parkinson disease: a randomized controlled trial. *Mov Disord*. 2007;22:2070-2076.

43 Schwarz R, Krauss O, Hinz A. Fatigue in the general population. *Onkologie*. 2003;26:140-144.

44 Brown RG, Dittner A, Findley L, Wessely SC. The Parkinson fatigue scale. *Parkinsonism Relat Disord*. 2005;11:49-55.

45 Hagell P, Rosblom T, Pålhagen S. A Swedish version of the 16-item Parkinson fatigue scale (PFS-16). *Acta Neurol Scand*. 2012;125:288-292.

46 Kummer A, Scalzo P, Cardoso F, Teixeira AL. Evaluation of fatigue in Parkinson's disease using the Brazilian version of Parkinson's Fatigue Scale. *Acta Neurol Scand*. 2011;123:130-136.

47 Rascol O, Fitzer-Attas CJ, Hauser R, et al. A double-blind, delayed-start trial of rasagiline in Parkinson's disease (the ADAGIO study): prespecified and post-hoc analyses of the need for additional therapies, changes in UPDRS scores, and non-motor outcomes. *Lancet Neurol*. 2011;10:415-423.

48 Morita A, Okuma Y, Kamei S, et al. Pramipexole reduces the prevalence of fatigue in patients with Parkinson's disease. *Intern Med*. 2011;50:2163-2168.

7. Cognition and neuropsychiatric symptoms

This section reviews scales that evaluate cognitive dysfunction and neuropsychiatric symptoms such as behavioural problems, psychotic complications, depression, and apathy. Behavioural problems and psychotic complications (eg, psychomotor agitation and hallucinations), are important sources of caregiver burden, and frequently constitute a reason for institutionalization. In Parkinson's disease (PD), depression is very prevalent and is a significant determinant of both patient's and caregiver's quality of life.

Scales for Outcomes in Parkinson's Disease-Cognition (SCOPA-Cog) (Figure 7.1) [1]	
Description of scale	
Overview	For evaluation of cognitive deficits in PD
	Ten items, assessing visual and verbal memory, delayed recall, executive and visuospatial functions and attention. Maximum score is 43, reflecting good cognitive status
	Time to complete the scale: 10 to 20 minutes
	Rated by a health professional
	Specific for PD
Copyright?	Owned by SCOPA-Propark Study
How can the scale be obtained?	The scale is available free of charge with permission of the authors in the website: www.scopa-propark.eu
Clinimetric properties of scale in patients with PD	
Feasibility	It has been applied to patients in all stages [1–3]
	Lower scores in patients with more advanced PD [1]
Dimensionality	Items correspond to cognitive domains. Rasch analysis has proved its unidimensionality [4]
Acceptability	Full range of scores was not covered in Spanish and Brazilian validation studies [2,3]. Score distribution was close to a normal distribution [5]
	Scoring system in some items should be modified [4]
	Floor and ceiling effects present in some items and domains [2]
	Skewness within acceptable limits [3,5]
Reliability	Person Separation Index, an estimate of reliability following Rasch analysis, reached 0.83 for SCOPA-Cog total score [4], indicating that at least 3 ability groups can be reliably distinguished
	Internal consistency: satisfactory [1–3,5]
	Inter-rater reliability: not tested
	Test-retest reliability: satisfactory results for total score, although lower for some items [1,3]

© Springer Healthcare 2014

P. Martinez-Martin et al., *Guide to Assessment Scales in Parkinson's Disease*,
DOI: 10.1007/978-1-907673-88-7_7

Validity	Content validity: those items that best discriminated between patients and controls were selected [1]; however, content validity has been criticized [6]
	Convergent: high correlation with Mini Mental State Examination (MMSE), MiniMental Parkinson (MMP), Cambridge Cognition Examination (CAMCOG), and Clinical Impression of Severity Index for Parkinson's Disease (CISI-PD) [1–3,5]. Lower with Hoehn & Yahr Staging Scale (HY), Short Portable Mental Status Questionnaire (SMPSQ) and other clinical scales
	Known-groups: SCOPA-Cog total score significantly decreased as HY stage, age and disease duration increased and MMSE scores decreased [1–3,5]
	SCOPA-Cog distinguished between patients and controls [1] and between patients with PD with and without dementia [7]
	Predictive: a cutoff of ≤19 points indicates dementia [2]
Responsiveness & Interpretability	Standard error of measurement (SEM) and smallest real difference have been estimated [2,3,5]
	Men and women' scores are similar [1] but items one (immediate word recall) and ten (delayed word recall) displayed differential item functioning (DIF) by age, and item two (digits backward) DIF by sex and age [4]
Cross-cultural Adaptations & Others	Versions available in English, Spanish [2], Portuguese [3] and Dutch (www.scopa-propark.eu)
Overall impression	
Advantages	Short; acceptable, reliable and valid scale; specific for PD cognitive deficits [6]; full validation studies [1–3], including Rasch analysis [4]
Disadvantages	Mainly assesses frontal-subcortical cognitive defects; content validity and responsiveness may be questioned [6]

Parkinson's Disease Cognitive Rating Scale (PD-CRS) [8]	
Description of scale	
Overview	For assessment of whole spectrum of cognitive functions over the course of PD [8]
	Includes seven tasks assessing frontal-subcortical functions (score range: 0 to 114) and two tasks assessing instrumental-cortical functions (0 to 20). Total score range is 0 to 134. Higher scores reflect better cognitive functioning
	Time to complete the scale: mean of 17 minutes [6]
	Rater: care professional
	Generic scale
Copyright?	Public domain
How can the scale be obtained?	It can be obtained through the original publication [8]
Clinimetric properties of scale in patients with PD	
Feasibility	Specifically designed for PD
	The scale has been applied to patients with PD of all levels of severity [9] and can significantly distinguish between cognitively intact patients with PD and patients with PD with mild cognitive impairment (MCI) or dementia (PDD) [6]

Dimensionality	The scale includes two types of tasks and corresponding scores (cortical vs. subcortical), but its structure has not been formally tested
Acceptability	No floor or ceiling effect s in the total score; ceiling effect present in subcortical score. Skewness in total and subscales scores [9]
Reliability	Internal consistency: satisfactory [8,9]
	Inter-rater and test-retest reliability: high [8]
Validity	Content validity: not formally tested [8]
	Convergent: high correlation coefficients between PD-CRS and MMSE, SCOPA-Cog, and Addenbrooke's Cognitive Examination-Revised (ACE-R) [9,10]
	Known-groups: significant differences in PD-CRS scores between cognitively intact patients with PD, patients with PD with MCI or PDD [8], education levels, and CISI-PD severity level [9]
	Predictive: a cut-off score of ≤64 has been established for PDD [8]
Responsiveness & Interpretability	SEM has been calculated [9]. Authors estimate that instrumental-cortical items in the PC-CRS may be especially useful in sensitively detect mild PDD and those non-demented patients with PD with instrumental-cortical cognitive defects [8]
	No significant differences in PD-CRS scores by sex but older people showed significant lower scores [9]
Cross-cultural Adaptations & Others	No translations available
Overall impression	
Advantages	Appropriate validation process; discriminates between cognitively intact and MCI and PDD
Disadvantages	Lack of data on responsiveness

Montreal Cognitive Assessment (MoCA) [11]	
Description of scale	
Overview	Assessment of mild cognitive impairment in general population [11]
	Composed by 12 items assessing short-term memory recall, visuospatial abilities, executive functions, attention, concentration and working memory, language, and orientation. Maximum score is 30 points, with higher scores indicating better performance
	Time to complete the scale: 10 minutes [11]
	Rater: health professional
	Generic validated in PD [12–16]
Copyright?	Public domain
How can the scale be obtained?	The scale can be obtained from the website: www.mocatest.org/
	For commercial or research use, written permission should be granted from the authors

Clinimetric properties of scale in patients with PD

Feasibility	PD associated motor impairment does not affect MoCA performance [14]
	Successfully applied to patients with PD of all stages of severity [13]. Patients in higher HY stages showed lower MoCA scores [13,14]
Dimensionality	Items are grouped into subscales, but the scales' structure has not been tested
Acceptability	Range of scores for PD: 6 to 28 [13], 12 to 30 [15]
	No ceiling effect [13]
Reliability	Internal consistency: not tested in PD
	Inter-rater and test-retest reliability in patients with PD: satisfactory [13]
Validity	Content validity: not tested. Item selection process was based on the clinical intuition of the authors and on the performance of items [11]
	Convergent: high correlation coefficient with MMSE [13]
	Known-groups: significant differences in patients with PD grouped by HY stages [13], cognitive status [14,16]
	Predictive: cutoff of 24/25 for dementia; 26/27 for MCI [15]
Responsiveness & Interpretability	A longitudinal study reported that MoCA did not change significantly over time, suggesting that MoCA may be more sensitive for detecting early cognitive deficits [17]
	Older people and men scored lower in MoCA [14]. DIF by sex or age has not been analyzed
	Normative data are available from the website: www.mocatest.org/
Cross-cultural Adaptations & Others	Translated into 22 languages. Available through the website: www.mocatest.org/
Overall impression	
Advantages	Sensitive to mild cognitive deficits in PD; fulfills the Movement Disorders Society (MDS) Task Force criteria for cognitive screening instruments in PD [18]
Disadvantages	The naming task has not been properly validated; cutoff values for dementia and MCI are not firmly established [18]; lacks a full clinimetric validation in PD

Neuropsychiatric Inventory (NPI) [19,20]	
Description of scale	
Overview	The NPI is a structured interview developed to assess behavioral problems in patients with dementia. The first version included 10 items [19], and subsequently 2 items were added: sleep and appetite disturbances [20]. The 12-item version is the one currently used. There is a probe question for each symptom and behavior; if endorsed, a score for severity (1 to 3) and frequency (1 to 4) is obtained and multiplied to get the score for each domain; higher values indicate worse functioning
	The NPI interview is made by a trained rater to a caregiver knowledgeable of the patient, and it takes approximately 15–30 minutes to administer [21]. There is also a questionnaire version (NPI-Q), completed by the caregiver and reviewed by the clinician, and a Nursing Home version for institutional settings (NPI-NH). Although used in PD [22], this scale was not specifically developed for PD
Copyright?	Copyright owned by Jeffrey Cummings, originator of the scale
How can the scale be obtained?	It may be obtained through http://npitest.net/about-npi.html
Clinimetric properties of scale in patients with PD	
Feasibility	The NPI questions are appropriate for the PD population, and the NPI is applicable across the PD stages
Dimensionality	There is no study on the dimensionality of the NPI applied to PD
Acceptability	Floor and ceiling effects, as well the distribution skewness in patients with PD, are not reported
Reliability	There is no information about internal consistency or test-retest reliability in PD. Inter-rater reliability was low in one study reporting on level of agreement between patient and caregiver [23], but another study reported high correlations between these two ratings (0.94 to 0.98) [24]
Validity	Content validity is estimated to be high. It presents moderate-to-high convergent validity with related scales: similar items of NPI and SCOPA-Psychiatric Complications (SCOPA-PC) [25], and Clinical Global Impression–Severity Scale (CGI-S) [26]; the NPI Apathy section and the Lille Apathy Rating Scale (LARS) [27]; quality of life and the Parkinson's Disease Questionnaire – 39 items (PDQ-39) [28]; and caregiver distress [29]
	Known-groups validity: the NPI was able to significantly differentiate patients with PD and healthy controls [30] or Alzheimer's disease patients [31]
Responsiveness & Interpretability	The NPI has been used in several PD medication trials, and either the total or specific domain scores showed adequate sensitivity to change in most studies [32–36], but not all [37,38]
	Valid for both sexes and all ages
Cross-cultural adaptations & Others	Translated into a large number of languages, although not all versions underwent a full linguistic validation process

Overall impression	
Advantages	Classified by the MDS-Task force as a 'recommended' scale to assess psychosis in PD; especially useful in cognitively impaired patients with PD [21]. NPI anxiety and apathy sections met the criteria for 'suggested' scales for PD anxiety and apathy, respectively [39,40]
Disadvantages	Many clinimetric features unknown in PD population [21]

Scales for Outcomes in Parkinson's Disease – Psychiatric Complications (SCOPAPC) [25] This scale is based on a previous version, the modified Parkinson Psychosis Rating Scale (mPPRS) [41,42], which is very similar to the SCOPA-PC, with one item less	
Description of scale	
Overview	The SCOPA-PC aims to assess psychotic and compulsive complications in PD [25]. It is formed of seven items, answered in a scale from 0 (absent) to 3 (severe). A short description is provided for scoring. In addition, interview questions are offered as a guide to help the clinician gather information from the patient and caregiver. The total sumscore ranges from 0 to 21, with higher scores indicating greater impairment. Two subscores have been used, by adding the compulsive items (Sexual preoccupation and Compulsive behavior) or psychotic symptoms (rest of the items) [43] Time to complete the scale: 5 to 10 minutes [25] Time frame: the previous month Specifically developed for PD
Copyright?	The SCOPA-PC, Parkinson Psychosis Rating Scale (PPRS), and mPPRS and are public domain scales [25,41,42]
How can the scale be obtained?	The SCOPA-PC is available at: www.scopa-propark.eu/
Clinimetric properties of scale in patients with PD	
Feasibility	The mPPRS questions were judged as being relevant by a panel of six experts (neurologists or psychiatrists) [42]. The SCOPA-PC is applicable across all PD stages
Dimensionality	Exploratory factor analysis of the mPPRS indicates the presence of a single factor, excluding item 6 (Sexuality) [42]
Acceptability	The mPPRS total score displayed a strong floor effect; skewness and kurtosis were also high [42]. SCOPA-PC items did not show a ceiling effect [25]
Reliability	Internal consistency was acceptable for the different versions of the scale [41,42]. Inter-rater and test-retest reliability of the SCOPA-PC were satisfactory [25]
Validity	Content validity of the mPPRS is adequate, as defined by a panel of experts [42]. Convergent validity with cognition measures is low and moderate-to-high with other psychosis measures, and shows inconsistent results with PD global severity [25,41,42]. The SCOPA-PC correlates at a moderate level with PD non-motor symptoms [44]. Known-groups validity was significant with HY staging (mPPRS) and medication regimen (mPPRS and SCOPA-PC) [25,41,43], as well as level of visual misperceptions [45] and presence of genetic mutations [46]

Responsiveness & Interpretability	The SCOPA-PC showed sensitivity to change in a two-year follow-up study [47]
Cross-cultural Adaptations & Others	The original PPRS was developed in Israel, and published in English [41]. The mPPRS Spanish version was the result of a translation-back translation process, which was then adjusted to Spanish for Ecuador, Paraguay and Argentina, and translated to Portuguese for Brazil and Guarani [42]. The SCOPA-PC is available in English, Dutch [25], Portuguese (Brazil), Spanish, and German (SCOPA scales website: www.scopa-propark.eu/)
Overall impression	
Advantages	Specifically developed for PD, the PPRS was classified as a 'suggested' scale for assessment of PD psychosis [21]
Disadvantages	Criticized for confusing anchors and multidimensional items [21]

Hamilton Depression Rating Scale (HAM-D) [48]	
Description of scale	
Overview	The HAM-D was developed to assess depressive symptoms of patients diagnosed with depression [48]. It is formed of 21 items, the first 17 of which contribute to the total score. The 17-item HAM-D, excluding the last 4 items, is frequently used. Different items have different response scales: 10 items are scored from 0 to 4, 9 items from 0 to 2 items, and 2 from 0 to 3. A higher score indicates more severe depression. The HAM-D is administered by a trained rater, and a structured interview guide is available [49] Time frame is the week prior to assessment Time to complete the scale: 15 minutes [50] The HAM-D is a generic scale that has been validated and is commonly used in PD [50,51]
Copyright?	Public domain
How can the scale be obtained?	http ://healthnet.umassmed.edu/mhealth/HAMD.pdf
Clinimetric properties of scale in patients with PD	
Feasibility	Questions are appropriate for PD population. Applicable across PD stages
Dimensionality	Dimensionality of the HAM-D in a psychiatric population has been questioned [52]. There is no information about the HAM-D structure when applied to patients with PD
Acceptability	Not assessed in PD
Reliability	Not assessed in PD. For the general or psychiatric population, the internal consistency of the HAM-D is adequate, and inconsistent results have been found for inter-rater and test-retest reliability [53]

Validity	HAM-D has been criticized for being conceptually flawed [53]. The HAM-D showed a significant association with extrapyramidal signs [54], functional ability [55], quality of life [28], suicidal ideation [56], and social anxiety [57] in patients with PD. It showed moderate-to-high convergent validity with other depression scales applied to patients with PD [51,55,58], and adequate concurrent validity with the *Diagnostic and Statistical Manual of Mental Disorders, Fourth Edition (DSM-IV)* criteria [59]
	The scale significantly discriminated between groups of patients with PD defined by level of physical and cognitive impairment [55], patients who have received deep brain stimulation (vs. controls) [60], and patients with PD vs. healthy controls [61]
	Different studies propose specific cut-off scores for patients with PD: 9/10 or 11/12 for screening purposes; 15/16 or 13/14 for diagnostic purposes [51,59]
Responsiveness & Interpretability	This scale was sensitive to change in clinical trials in patients with PD [62–71]
	The HAM-D is valid for both sexes and across all PD stages
Cross-cultural Adaptations & Others	The HAM-D has been translated in most European and Asian languages [50]
Overall impression	
Advantages	Useful, valid scale for screening purposes; 'recommended' scale for assessing severity of depressive symptoms [50]; self-rated
Disadvantages	Limited information about its clinimetric properties in PD and several flaws identified [53]; over-representation of somatic symptoms, some of them overlapping with PD cardinal manifestations [50]

Beck Depression Inventory (BDI) [72]	
Description of scale	
Overview	The BDI is formed of 21 items, rated in a 4-point scale form 0 (least severe) to 3 (most severe). The scale was designed to be applied through interview [72], although it is most usually self-completed. Time to complete the scale is 5 to 10 minutes (self-completed) to 15 minutes (interview) [50]. The most widely used version is the revised Beck Depression Inventory (BDI-IA), where the time frame was lengthened from current time to 'last week', and some items and descriptors were reworded. A second, less used version, the BDI-II, refers to the 2 weeks prior to assessment [73]
	Generic scale, but appropriate for use in PD [50]
Copyright?	Owned by Psychcorp
How can the scale be obtained?	Through Psychcorp (TM), part of Pearson Education
Clinimetric properties of scale in patients with PD	
Feasibility	Questions are appropriate for PD. Applicable across most PD stages. Patients with cognitive impairment might have difficulty in understanding the questions (ie, the anchors are quite long)
Dimensionality	Exploratory factor analysis of the BDI applied to PD indicates the presence of two factors: cognitive-affective and somatic [74]
Acceptability	When applied to PD, five BDI items show a floor effect, and none shows a ceiling effect [74]

Reliability	Internal consistency of the BDI applied to PD is adequate (Cronbach's alpha: 0.88) [74,75]. Test-retest reliability was adequate for all but two items and for the total score [74]
Validity	Face validity is adequate: most BDI items correspond to DSM-IV criteria for depression [50]
	The BDI discriminates between patients with PD and controls [74], and patients with PD by depression status [76]. The BDI shows a high convergent validity with other depression scales and low-to-moderate associations with PD stage, physical impairment, motor function, and UPDRS (Unified Parkinson's Disease Rating Scale) humor item [76]. Concurrent validity with DSM-IV is fair [51]
	Proposed cut-off scores: from 8/9 to 17/18 [74,76–78]. Low cut-off values are appropriate for screening and high values for diagnostic purposes [77]
Responsiveness & Interpretability	BDI was sensitive to change in several clinical trial in PD [63,66,79]
	The smallest real difference in PD was 3.3 points (total BDI) [74]
	Valid for both sexes and across ages
Cross-cultural Adaptations & Others	Translated and culturally validated in many European, Asian, and African languages [80]
Overall impression	
Advantages	Widely used; satisfactory clinimetric properties in PD; useful for screening and severity assessment; appropriate cutoff scores. BDI has been classified as valid for screening purposes, and 'recommended' for diagnostic purposes [50]
Disadvantages	In spite of including many somatic symptoms, BDI discriminates between groups of patients with PD with and without depression; there is no information about the clinimetric properties of the BDI-II in PD; many cut-off scores proposed

Hospital Anxiety and Depression Scale (HADS) [81]	
Description of scale	
Overview	The HADS was designed to screen for anxiety and depression in medical outpatients from a general hospital [81] and, therefore, it does not include somatic items. It is formed by 2 subscales: Anxiety and Depression, each with 7 items scored from 0 (least severe) to 3 (more severe). Anxiety and depression items alternate, and anxiety items are even-numbered. A sumscore is calculated for each subscale, although a total sumscore can also be used. The depression items focus mainly on anhedonia
	Time frame is one week [81] and it takes a few minutes to complete. The scale is self-completed. This is a generic scale, but there are several validation studies in PD [58,82–85]
Copyright?	Owned by GL assessment
How can the scale be obtained?	http://www.gl-assessment.co.uk/

Clinimetric properties of scale in patients with PD

Feasibility	Questions are appropriate for PD, and it is applicable across PD stages [50,39]
Dimensionality	There is some debate about the scale's unidimensionality, and contradictory results have been found [85]. The total score can be used as a measure of general distress, and there is evidence that the anxiety subscale is unidimensional [84]
Acceptability	The total score follows a normal distribution [82,84]. Studies report absence of floor or ceiling effects for the subscales and total score [82,83,85]
Reliability	Internal consistency is adequate [82,83,85], with only one study reporting a Cronbach's alpha value of 0.69 for the depression subscale [85]. Test-retest reliability is satisfactory [82,85]
Validity	Face validity is moderate [39,50]. Internal validity is adequate (correlation 0.61 to 0.62 between subscales) [82,83,85]. The HADS shows adequate convergent validity with PD quality of life measures [82], but the HADS anxiety subscale showed low-to-moderate correlations with other anxiety measures [85]. Correlation with age and PD duration was weak [82,83]
	Known-groups validity was supported by significant differences by clinical global impression of anxiety symptoms and type of anxiety disorder [85], as well as disease stage, severity, and PD duration [83]. The HADS anxiety subscale was not correlated with degree of disability or severity of motor symptoms [86]
	Predictive validity was established against the HAM-D and clinical global impression of anxiety symptoms, with suggested cut-off scores of 10/11 [43] or 13/14 [85] for the total score, and 6/7 for the HADS anxiety subscale [85]
Responsiveness & Interpretability	Sensitive to change after unilateral pallidotomy [86], deep brain stimulation [87], and sertraline treatment [88], but not after rehabilitation [89]
	Estimated minimal important difference (MID): total scale, 5.9; anxiety subscale, 4.2; depression subscale, 3.6 [85]
	Valid for both sexes and all ages. One PD study analyzed differential item functioning by sex and all items were free from bias [84]
Cross-cultural Adaptations & Others	The HADS is available in many languages

Overall impression

Advantages	Quick self-administered scale, with several validation studies in PD, using both Rasch analysis and classic psychometric methods [58,82–85]; in a comparison of three anxiety scales in PD, the HADS was considered to be the most appropriate [86]. 'Suggested' scale to screen for anxiety [39] and 'moderately suitable' to screen for depression in patients with PD [50]
Disadvantages	Questionable face validity, since both subscales do not include some relevant aspects of anxiety and depression; the scale's dimensionality is controversial

Montgomery-Åsberg Depression Rating Scale (MADRS) [90]	
Description of scale	
Overview	The MADRS is a depression rating scale designed to be sensitive to depression treatment effects [90]. It is formed by 10 items, rated on a 0 (normal or not present) to 6 (most severe) scale. Anchors are defined for even steps of the response scale. The scale is rated by a clinician who should have some clinical experience with depression. No time frame is specified
	Time to complete the scale: approximately 15 minutes
	Generic depression scale, with some validation studies in PD [51,78]
Copyright?	The MADRS is copyrighted by Stuart Montgomery, M.D. Permission is granted by the author to reproduce the scale on a website for clinicians to use in their practice and for use in non-industry studies
How can the scale be obtained?	Available in several Web pages such as www.outcometracker.org/library/MADRS.pdf
Clinimetric properties of scale in patients with PD	
Feasibility	Questions are appropriate for PD, and the scale is applicable across PD stages
Dimensionality	Not assessed in PD
Acceptability	There is no information about the score distribution and floor/ceiling effects in PD
Reliability	To date, there are no studies that report information about the reliability of the MADRS in PD
Validity	Face validity is satisfactory. It covers almost all DSM-IV aspects of depression
	The MADRS was associated with psychosocial burden on spouses of patients with PD [91], changes in sleep [92], quality of life [93,94], risk of care dependency [95], and neuropsychiatric symptoms [96]. Dopaminergic activity was associated with the MADRS total score [97]. Able to differentiate between groups defined by the presence of pain [98] and dementia [99], HY stage [99], depression diagnosis [100], and PD patient versus. controls [101]. The following adjusted cut-off values for PD [102] were suggested: 14/15 for screening [51] and 17/18 for diagnosis [51,78]
Responsiveness & Interpretability	Sensitive to change in several treatment studies [92,103–106]
Cross-cultural Adaptations & Others	It is available in several European and Asian languages [50]
Overall impression	
Advantages	Classified as a valid scale for screening, and 'recommended' for diagnostic purposes [50]; sensitive to change in PD [92,103–106]
Disadvantages	Few validation studies in PD, with some clinimetric attributes unexplored in this population; must be completed by rater with experience

Geriatric Depression Scale (GDS) [107]	
Description of scale	
Overview	The GDS was developed as a self-rating screening scale for depression in older adults. It was originally developed with 30 items (GDS-30), and 3 years later a shorter, 15-item version (GDS-15) was published [108]. In both versions, items are answered by circling yes or no, and higher total scores indicate increased severity of depression
	Time frame: the week prior to assessment
	Self-reported scale, although scores can be recorded by an observer
	Time to complete the scale: 15 minutes for the GDS-30; 10 minutes for the GDS-15 [109]. Generic scale for the geriatric population. It has been partially validated in PD [58,110]
Copyright?	The GDS-15 and GDS-30 are in the public domain
How can the scale be obtained?	www.stanford.edu/~yesavage/GDS.html
Clinimetric properties of scale in patients with PD	
Feasibility	Questions are appropriate for PD and the GDS is applicable across all PD stages. Applicable to patients aged 55 years and older of both sexes
Dimensionality	A three-factor structure was found for the GDS-15 when applied to patients with PD [111]
Acceptability	Unknown
Reliability	Internal consistency of the GDS-30 was high (Cronbach's alpha: 0.92) [112]
Validity	The GDS items were developed to maximize discrimination between depressed and non-depressed older adults [107], and its face validity is satisfactory [50]
	The GDS-30 and GDS-15 showed a moderate-to-high convergent validity with the HAM-D [113] and Zung Self-Rating Depression Scale (ZSDS) [114]. The GDS-30 correlated at a moderate-to-high level with the BDI, HADS, HAM-D, and a visual analogue scale (VAS) for depression [58,76]. The GDS-15 showed low correlation coefficients with PD duration, severity, and functional capacity [76]
	The GDS-15 significantly differentiated between groups of patients with PD defined by disease severity and duration, and cognitive function [115]. Proposed GDS-15 cut-off is 5/6 for older patients with PD (above 75 years old) and 4/5 for younger ages [110,116]. Another study suggested 8/9 as a screening GDS-15 cut-off score [76]. Using the GDS-30, a cut-off of 10/11 was suggested as the most suitable for screening purposes, and 12/13 for diagnosis [58]. Another study with a smaller sample proposed different values [112]
Responsiveness & Interpretability	There are very few studies on the GDS sensitivity to change [117,118]
Cross-cultural Adaptations & Others	The GDS has been translated into many languages

Overall impression

Advantages	Valid scale for screening purposes in PD [50]; the GDS-30 and the GDS-15 showed best performance and efficiency for screening of depression in PD than other scales [76,119,120]
Disadvantages	For both GDS versions, there is no agreement about the best cut-off value to be used for diagnosis; more studies are needed about its clinimetric properties and the usefulness of the GDS in young patients with PD
Comments	Clinicians should be aware that the GDS does not include questions about suicide

Apathy Scale (AS) [121]

Description of scale

Overview	Assesses apathy in patients with PD
	Derived from the Marin's Apathy Scale [122], this scale is formed by 14 items, answered in a 0 to 3 Likert type scale, with a total sumscore. Higher scores indicate more severe apathy
	Time for administration: Not reported, but estimated as 5 to 10 minutes
	Time frame: Previous 4 weeks
	The examiner reads aloud the questions to the patient, who rates them. There is also a caregiver-rated version [123]
	This is a specific scale for PD
Copyright?	Public domain
How can the scale be obtained?	Available in several Web pages such as http://www.dementia-assessment.com.au/symptoms/

Clinimetric properties of scale in patients with PD

Feasibility	It was designed specifically for patients with PD. Not useful for patients with dementia or with very low insight into their apathy symptoms [40]
Dimensionality	Exploratory factor analysis indicates the presence of two factors (cognitive-behavioral aspects and general apathy) [124]. However, the total sumscore is usually used
Acceptability	No floor effect in patients without apathy [121]
Reliability	Adequate internal consistency, with Cronbach alpha rating from 0.69 to 0.90 [121,123,124]. Test-retest and inter-rater reliability are appropriate, although it was tested on limited group of patients [121,123]
Validity	Satisfactory face validity [40]
	Known-groups validity: significantly different apathy scores by severity of cognitive impairment [121]. Fair discriminant validity [124]
	High correlation coefficients with other apathy scales: LARS and BDI [125]
	Adequate criterion validity against the clinical impression used as a gold standard [121]
	Suggested cutoff scores: scores of 14 or higher indicate clinically meaningful apathy in PD [121], with a sensitivity of 100% and specificity of 66% [121]

Responsiveness & Interpretability	Sensitive to change by dopaminergic treatment and subtalamic nucleus stimulation [126–129]. No information available about precision or MID
Cross-cultural Adaptations & Others	Published studies reporting its use in several languages, such as French, English, Japanese, Italian, Polish, and Spanish
Overall impression	
Advantages	Easy to use; can be rated by the patient or caregiver; adequate reliability and validity; defined cut-off scores. The AS was 'recommended' for use in PD by the MDS-Task Force serving both as a screening and severity measure [40]
Disadvantages	Limited information about acceptability; limited use in patients with low insight or dementia [40]

Figure 7.1 Scales for Outcomes in Parkinson's Disease (SCOPA-Cog)

Memory and learning

1. Verbal recall

Ten words are repeatedly shown for at least 4 seconds, get the patient to read them out loud. The time allowed for recall is unlimited. Underline each word that has been named. When words are named that were not shown, no penalty is given. When a false answer is changed (eg, king into queen), it is correct.

Instruction: "Read the following 10 words aloud and try to remember as many as possible. After reading them all, name as many words as possible, the order of the words is not important".

10 words: Butter arm shore letter queen cabin pole ticket grass engine

(10 correct = 5; 8–9 correct = 4; 6–7 correct = 3; 5 correct = 2, 4 correct = 1; ≤ 3 correct= 0)
score /5

2. Digit span backward

Ask the patient to repeat a series of numbers backwards; the numbers are read out separately, 1 second per number; if incorrectly repeated, the alternative in the second column is presented. Continue until both the first and the alternative series are repeated incorrectly. Make sure the time interval between numbers stays the same. Read the numbers calmly and make sure the time between numbers is equal. Record the highest series that is repeated correctly at least once. Give an example: "If I say 2-7-3, than you say (3-7-2)"

backwards		score:
2-4	5-8	= 1
6-2-9	4-1-5	= 2
3-2-7-9	4-9-6-8	= 3
1-5-2-8-6	6-1-8-4-3	= 4
5-3-9-4-1-8	7-2-4-8-5-6	= 5
8-1-2-9-3-6-5	4-7-3-9-1-2-8	= 6
9-4-3-7-6-2-5-8	7-2-8-1-9-6-5-3	= 7

score /7

3. *Indicate cubes*
Point to the cubes in the order given below; the patient should copy this; do this slowly; the patient decides for himself with which hand he/she prefers. Indicate the cubes in the order as indicated. Observe carefully if the patient copies the order correctly. When a patient wants to correct a mistake, let him/her do the complete order again. This is not counted as a mistake. However, if the patient forgets the order and would like to see the order a second time, the researcher does not repeat the order again but starts with the next order.

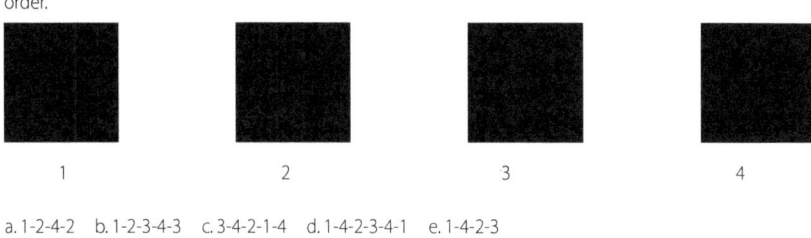

a. 1-2-4-2 b. 1-2-3-4-3 c. 3-4-2-1-4 d. 1-4-2-3-4-1 e. 1-4-2-3
score /5

Attention

4. *Counting backwards (30 to 0)*
Instruction: "Would you subtract 3 from 30, and subtract 3 again from the result, and continue until 0?".

Mistakes can be: the order, missing or not knowing a number, or not finishing off the series. Record the order of numbers named by the patient. If the patient asks where to start or how much to subtract, the researcher repeats the instructions but counts that as one mistake. If the patient makes a mistake but continues from that point to subtract three, it is only one mistake. If the patient stops the order and starts all over again, it is one mistake.

(0 mistakes = 2; 1 mistake = 1; ≥2 mistakes = 0)
score   /2

5. *Months backwards*
Instruction: "Name the months of the year in reverse order, starting with the last month of the year".

Mistakes are: the order, missing or not knowing the next month, or not finishing off the series. Underline the months that are named correctly. When a month is passed over, this is a mistake, even if the patient corrects it later on. If the patient stops the order and starts all over again, it is one mistake. If the patient starts naming the month forward, repeat the instructions and count it as one mistake.
Dec- Nov-Oct-Sept-Aug-July-June-May-April-March-Feb-Jan.

(0 mistakes = 2; 1 mistake = 1; ≥2 mistakes = 0)
score   / 2

Executive functions

6. Fist-edge-palm

1. Make a fist with ulnar side down, 2. Stretch fingers with ulnar side down 3. Stretch fingers with palm down; Practice 5 times together with the patient. The patient chooses which hand he/she prefers. Do it slowly and tell the patient to watch carefully and repeat what you are doing. Practice first 5 rounds, with verbal help, (eg, say Fist Stretch Palm aloud as you make each movement). Then tell the patient to make the movements alone.

Instructions: "Now it is your turn to make the three movements, fist-stretch-palm, 10 times in a row. You don't have to count, I will tell you when to stop".

Note the number of correct trios from a total of 10; Count carefully but not out loud. Every time a patient makes a wrong movement, count it as a mistake, even when the patient corrects it halfway.

(10 correct = 3; 9 correct = 2;, 8 correct = 1;≤7 correct = 0)

score   /3

7. Semantic fluency

Tell the patient to name as many animal as he/she knows in one minute. Note all answers that are given by the patient. No repetition or variations of words, such as lion-lioness, tiger-tigress; categories are allowed, (ie, bird and pigeon are both correct). Count the number of animals correctly named. The purpose is that the patient generates the animals actively, therefore no clues are allowed. When the patient asks whether, for instance, naming different types of birds is allowed, this may be confirmed. When the patient almost immediately says he/she does not know any more animals, try to stimulate the patient by saying "there is still a lot of time left," but do not give clues. When the patient starts naming things other than animals, do not correct the patient. Naming other things besides animals is not counted as an additional mistake.

(≥ 25 correct = 6; 20–24 = 5; 15–19 = 4, 10–14 = 3; 5-9 = 2; 1–4 = 1; 0=0)

number of animals correct

score   /6

Write down all animals named:

8. Dice

Use 2 cards, one with YES = EVEN, NO = ODD; one with YES = HIGHER, NO = LOWER. Put the correct card face up next to the explanation of the test and make sure that the other, irrelevant card is out of sight. The first round (situation 1) is not scored, and the patient is corrected if necessary.

Situation 1: YES = EVEN

Put the card "YES=EVEN, NO=ODD" on the table and leave it there during the test. Instruction: "Say YES for an even number on a dice and NO for an odd numbe. When you see a picture of a dice with an EVEN number of pips, I would like you to say YES, and NO when the number of pips is ODD".
Show the first two examples (3 even and 3 odd dices) and ask the patient "If you see one of these dice, do you say yes or no?" Tell the patient if the answer is correct or not. If the answer is not correct, explain why. It is important that the patient says YES or NO and not EVEN or ODD. Show the next two examples (with only one dice) and ask the patient "if you see this dice, do you say yes or no?" Tell the patient if the answer is correct or not. If the answer is not correct, explain why.
Then show the patient the following 10 dices. Correct the patient if the answer is wrong.

Situation 2: YES = HIGHER
With the card "example 1" (dice with 3 pips), the next condition starts. Put the card "YES=HIGHER, NO=LOWER" on the table and remove the former card.
Instruction: "Now, we change the test a little. When you see a picture of a dice that is higher than the dice on the page before, you say YES. When the dice is lower, you say NO".
Tell the patient you have an example (use example 1). "Try to remember this dice" (turn the page) "Is this YES or NO?" Tell the patient whether the answer is correct or not. If the answer is not correct, explain why. Continue with example 2 and say "now remember this dice" (turn the page) "Is this YES or NO?" Tell the patient if the answer is correct or not. If the answer is not correct, explain why.

Then start the test and show all 10 dice one after another. The first response counts and corrections are not allowed. Do NOT correct when a wrong answer is given. If a patient corrects a wrong answer, it is still counted as a mistake. If the patient asks for the instruction, the researcher explains but that is counted as one mistake.

(10 correct = 3; 9 correct = 2; 8 correct =1; ≤7 correct = 0)
number correct   /10
score   /3

Visuo-spatial functions

9. Assembling patterns
The patient is shown 5 incomplete patterns and has to choose 2 or 3 shapes out of 4 to 6 possible alternatives in order to complete the pattern. First practice with 2 figures.
Show the patient example A and give the instruction to choose the shapes that form the pattern. Tell the patient if the answer is correct or not. If the answer is not correct, explain why and give the correct solution. Repeat this with example B. Then show the 5 patterns. Do not tell the patient whether the answer is correct or not. There is no time limit. If the patient corrects a wrong answer, this is not counted as a mistake.
a.   b.   c.   d.   e.

score   /5

Memory

10. Delayed recall
Instruction: "Can you name as many as possible of the 10 words that you learned during the first test?"
Underline each word that has been named. When words are named that were not shown, no penalty is given. When a false answer is changed (eg, king into queen), it is correct.
10 words: butter arm shore letter queen cabin pole ticket grass engine

(10 correct = 5; 8–9 correct = 4; 6–7 correct = 3; 5 correct = 2; 4 correct = 1; ≤3 correct= 0)
number of correct words   /10
score   /5

Total COG score   /43

References

1   Marinus J, Visser M, Verwey NA, et al. Assessment of cognition in Parkinson's disease. *Neurology*. 2003;61:1222-1228.

2   Martínez-Martín P, Frades-Payo B, Rodríguez-Blázquez C, et al. [Psychometric attributes of Scales for Outcomes in Parkinson's Disease-Cognition (SCOPA-Cog), Castilian language]. *Rev Neurol*. 2008;47:337-343.

3   Carod-Artal FJ, Martínez-Martin P, Kummer W, Ribeiro L da S. Psychometric attributes of the SCOPA-COG Brazilian version. *Mov Disord*. 2008;23:81-87.

4   Forjaz MJ, Frades-Payo B, Rodriguez-Blazquez C, Ayala A, Martinez-Martin P. Should the SCOPA-COG be modified? A Rasch analysis perspective. *Eur J Neurol*. 2010;17:202-207.

5   Serrano-Dueñas M, Calero B, Serrano S, Serrano M, Coronel P. Metric properties of the mini-mental Parkinson and SCOPA-COG scales for rating cognitive deterioration in Parkinson's disease. *Mov Disord*. 2010;25:2555-2562.

6   Kulisevsky J, Pagonabarraga J. Cognitive impairment in Parkinson's disease: tools for diagnosis and assessment. *Mov Disord*. 2009;24:1103-1110.

7   Martinez-Martin P, Falup-Pecurariu C, Rodriguez-Blazquez C, et al. Dementia associated with Parkinson's disease: applying the Movement Disorder Society Task Force criteria. *Parkinsonism Relat Disord*. 2011;17:621-624.

8   Pagonabarraga J, Kulisevsky J, Llebaria G, García-Sánchez C, Pascual-Sedano B, Gironell A. Parkinson's disease-cognitive rating scale: a new cognitive scale specific for Parkinson's disease. *Mov Disord*. 2008;23:998-1005.

9   Martínez-Martín P, Prieto-Jurczynska C, Frades-Payo B. [Psychometric attributes of the Parkinson's Disease-Cognitive Rating Scale. An independent validation study]. *Rev Neurol*. 2009;49:393-398.

10 McColgan P, Evans JR, Breen DP, Mason SL, Barker RA, Williams-Gray CH. Addenbrooke's Cognitive Examination-Revised for mild cognitive impairment in Parkinson's disease. *Mov Disord*. 2012;27:1173-1177.

11 Nasreddine ZS, Phillips NA, Bédirian V, et al. The Montreal Cognitive Assessment, MoCA: a brief screening tool for mild cognitive impairment. *J Am Geriatr Soc*. 2005;53:695-699.

12 Zadikoff C, Fox SH, Tang-Wai DF, et al. A comparison of the mini mental state exam to the Montreal cognitive assessment in identifying cognitive deficits in Parkinson's disease. *Mov Disord*. 2008;23:297-299.

13 Gill DJ, Freshman A, Blender JA, Ravina B. The Montreal cognitive assessment as a screening tool for cognitive impairment in Parkinson's disease. *Mov Disord*. 2008;23:1043-1046.

14 Nazem S, Siderowf AD, Duda JE, et al. Montreal cognitive assessment performance in patients with Parkinson's disease with «normal» global cognition according to mini-mental state examination score. *J Am Geriatr Soc*. 2009;57:304-308.

15 Hoops S, Nazem S, Siderowf AD, et al. Validity of the MoCA and MMSE in the detection of MCI and dementia in Parkinson disease. *Neurology*. 2009;73:1738-1745.

16 Dalrymple-Alford JC, MacAskill MR, Nakas CT, et al. The MoCA: well-suited screen for cognitive impairment in Parkinson disease. *Neurology*. 2010;75:1717-1725.

17 Lessig S, Nie D, Xu R, Corey-Bloom J. Changes on brief cognitive instruments over time in Parkinson's disease. *Mov Disord*. 2012;27:1125-1128.

18 Chou KL, Amick MM, Brandt J, et al; for the Parkinson Study Group Cognitive/Psychiatric Working Group. A recommended scale for cognitive screening in clinical trials of Parkinson's disease. *Mov Disord*. 2010;25:2501-2507.

19 Cummings JL, Mega M, Gray K, Rosenberg-Thompson S, Carusi DA, Gornbein J. The Neuropsychiatric Inventory: comprehensive assessment of psychopathology in dementia. *Neurology*. 1994;44:2308-2314.

20 Cummings JL. The Neuropsychiatric Inventory: assessing psychopathology in dementia patients. *Neurology*. 1997;48(suppl 6):S10-S16.

21 Fernandez HH, Aarsland D, Fénelon G, et al. Scales to assess psychosis in Parkinson's disease: Critique and recommendations. *Mov Disord*. 2008;23:484-500.

22 Aarsland D, Brønnick K, Ehrt U, et al. Neuropsychiatric symptoms in patients with Parkinson's disease and dementia: frequency, profile and associated care giver stress. *J Neurol Neurosurg Psychiatr*. 2007;78:36-42.

23 McKinlay A, Grace RC, Dalrymple-Alford JC, Anderson TJ, Fink J, Roger D. Neuropsychiatric problems in Parkinson's disease: comparisons between self and caregiver report. *Aging Ment Health*. 2008;12:647-653.

24 Stella F, Banzato CE, Quagliato EM, Viana MA, Christofoletti G. Psychopathological features in patients with Parkinson's disease and related caregivers' burden. *Int J Geriatr Psychiatry*. 2009;24:1158-1165.

25 Visser M, Verbaan D, van Rooden SM, Stiggelbout AM, Marinus J, van Hilten JJ. Assessment of psychiatric complications in Parkinson's disease: The SCOPA-PC. *Mov Disord*. 2007;22:2221-2228.

26 Chou KL, Messing S, Oakes D, Feldman PD, Breier A, Friedman JH. Drug-induced psychosis in Parkinson disease: phenomenology and correlations among psychosis rating instruments. *Clin Neuropharmacol*. 2005;28:215-219.

27 Drijgers RL, Dujardin K, Reijnders JS, Defebvre L, Leentjens AF. Validation of diagnostic criteria for apathy in Parkinson's disease. *Parkinsonism Relat Disord*. 2010;16:656-660.

28 Gómez-Esteban JC, Tijero B, Somme J, et al. Impact of psychiatric symptoms and sleep disorders on the quality of life of patients with Parkinson's disease. *J Neurol*. 2011;258:494-499.

29 D'Amelio M, Terruso V, Palmeri B, et al. Predictors of caregiver burden in partners of patients with Parkinson's disease. *Neurol Sci*. 2009;30:171-174.

30 Aarsland D, Brønnick K, Alves G, et al. The spectrum of neuropsychiatric symptoms in patients with early untreated Parkinson's disease. *J Neurol Neurosurg Psychiatry*. 2009;80:928-930.

31 Aarsland D, Cummings JL, Larsen JP. Neuropsychiatric differences between Parkinson's disease with dementia and Alzheimer's disease. *Int J Geriatr Psychiatry*. 2001;16:184-191.

32 Juncos JL, Roberts VJ, Evatt ML, et al. Quetiapine improves psychotic symptoms and cognition in Parkinson's disease. *Mov Disord*. 2004;19:29-35.

33 Giménez-Roldán S, Navarro E, Mateo D. [Effects of quetiapine at low doses on psychosis motor disability and stress of the caregiver in patients with Parkinson's disease]. *Rev Neurol*. 2003;36:401-404.

34 Rocha FL, Hara C, Ramos MG, et al. An exploratory open-label trial of ziprasidone for the treatment of behavioral and psychological symptoms of dementia. *Dement Geriatr Cogn Disord*. 2006;22:445-448.

35 Kawanabe T, Yoritaka A, Shimura H, Oizumi H, Tanaka S, Hattori N. Successful treatment with Yokukansan for behavioral and psychological symptoms of Parkinsonian dementia. *Prog Neuropsychopharmacol Biol Psychiatry*. 2010;34:284-287.

36 Merims D, Balas M, Peretz C, Shabtai H, Giladi N. Rater-blinded, prospective comparison: quetiapine versus clozapine for Parkinson's disease psychosis. *Clin Neuropharmacol*. 2006;29:331-337.

37 Tariot PN, Schneider L, Katz IR, et al. Quetiapine treatment of psychosis associated with dementia: a double-blind, randomized, placebo-controlled clinical trial. *Am J Geriatr Psychiatry*. 2006;14:767-776.

38 De Gaspari D, Siri C, Landi A, et al. Clinical and neuropsychological follow up at 12 months in patients with complicated Parkinson's disease treated with subcutaneous apomorphine infusion or deep brain stimulation of the subthalamic nucleus. *J Neurol Neurosurg Psychiatr*. 2006;77:450-453.

39 Leentjens AFG, Dujardin K, Marsh L, et al. Anxiety rating scales in Parkinson's disease: critique and recommendations. *Mov Disord*. 2008;23:2015-2025.

40 Leentjens AFG, Dujardin K, Marsh L, et al. Apathy and anhedonia rating scales in Parkinson's disease: critique and recommendations. *Mov Disord*. 2008;23:2004-2014.

41 Friedberg G, Zoldan J, Weizman A, Melamed E. Parkinson Psychosis Rating Scale: a practical instrument for grading psychosis in Parkinson's disease. *Clin Neuropharmacol*. 1998;21:280-284.

42 Virués-Ortega J, Rodríguez-Blázquez C, Micheli F, Carod-Artal FJ, Serrano-Dueñas M, Martínez-Martín P. Cross-cultural evaluation of the modified Parkinson Psychosis Rating Scale across disease stages. *Mov Disord*. 2010;25:1391-1398.

43 Verbaan D, van Rooden SM, Visser M, Marinus J, Emre M, van Hilten JJ. Psychotic and compulsive symptoms in Parkinson's disease. *Mov Disord*. 2009;24:738-744.

44 Martinez-Martin P, Rodriguez-Blazquez C, Abe K, et al. International study on the psychometric attributes of the non-motor symptoms scale in Parkinson disease. *Neurology*. 2009;73:1584-1591.

45 Shine JM, Halliday GH, Carlos M, Naismith SL, Lewis SJ. Investigating visual misperceptions in Parkinson's disease: A novel behavioral paradigm. *Mov Disord*. 2012;27:500-505.

46 Macedo MG, Verbaan D, Fang Y, et al. Genotypic and phenotypic characteristics of Dutch patients with early onset Parkinson's disease. *Mov Disord*. 2009;24:196-203.

47 Visser M, Verbaan D, van Rooden S, Marinus J, van Hilten J, Stiggelbout A. A Longitudinal Evaluation of Health-Related Quality of Life of Patients with Parkinson's Disease. *Value Health*. 2009;12:392-396.

48 Hamilton M. A Rating Scale for Depression. *J Neurol Neurosurg Psychiatry*. 1960;23:56-62.

49 Williams JBW. A Structured Interview Guide for the Hamilton Depression Rating Scale. *Arch Gen Psychiatry*. 1988;45:742-747.

50 Schrag A, Barone P, Brown RG, et al. Depression rating scales in Parkinson's disease: critique and recommendations. *Mov Disord*. 2007;22:1077-1092.

51 Leentjens AF, Verhey FR, Lousberg R, Spitsbergen H, Wilmink FW. The validity of the Hamilton and Montgomery-Åsberg depression rating scales as screening and diagnostic tools for depression in Parkinson's disease. *Int J Geriatr Psychiatry*. 2000;15:644-649.

52 Licht RW, Qvitzau S, Allerup P, Bech P. Validation of the Bech-Rafaelsen Melancholia Scale and the Hamilton Depression Scale in patients with major depression; is the total score a valid measure of illness severity? *Acta Psychiatr Scand*. 2005;111:144-149.

53 Bagby RM, Ryder AG, Schuller DR, Marshall MB. The Hamilton Depression Rating Scale: has the gold standard become a lead weight? *Am J Psychiatry*. 2004;161:2163-2177.

54 Starkstein SE, Petracca G, Chemerinski E, et al. Depression in classic versus akinetic-rigid Parkinson's disease. *Mov Disord*. 1998;13:29-33.

55 Starkstein SE, Preziosi TJ, Bolduc PL, Robinson RG. Depression in Parkinson's disease. *J Nerv Ment Dis*. 1990;178:27-31.

56 Kummer A, Cardoso F, Teixeira AL. Suicidal ideation in Parkinson's disease. *CNS Spectr*. 2009;14:431-436.

57 Kummer A, Cardoso F, Teixeira AL. Frequency of social phobia and psychometric properties of the Liebowitz social anxiety scale in Parkinson's disease. *Mov Disord*. 2008;23:1739-1743.

58 Mondolo F, Jahanshahi M, Granà A, Biasutti E, Cacciatori E, Di Benedetto P. The validity of the hospital anxiety and depression scale and the geriatric depression scale in Parkinson's disease. *Behav Neurol*. 2006;17:109-115.

59 Naarding P, Leentjens AFG, Van Kooten F, Verhey FRJ. Disease-specific properties of the Rating Scale for Depression in patients with stroke, Alzheimer's dementia, and Parkinson's disease. *J Neuropsychiatry Clin Neurosci*. 2002;14:329-334.

60 Fassino S, Abbate Daga G, Gramaglia C, et al. Novelty-seeking in Parkinson's disease after deep brain stimulation of the subthalamic nucleus: a case-control study. *Psychosomatics*. 2010;51:62-67.

61 Uluduz D, Ertürk O, Kenangil G, et al. Apraxia in Parkinson's disease and multiple system atrophy. *Eur J Neurol*. 2010;17:413-418.

62 Fetoni V, Soliveri P, Monza D, Testa D, Girotti F. Affective symptoms in multiple system atrophy and Parkinson's disease: response to levodopa therapy. *J Neurol Neurosurg Psychiatry*. 1999;66:541-544.

63 Fava M, Rosenbaum JF, Kolsky AR, et al. Open study of the catechol-O-methyltransferase inhibitor tolcapone in major depressive disorder. *J Clin Psychopharmacol*. 1999;19:329-335.

64 Pintor L, Baillès E, Valldeoriola F, Tolosa E, Martí MJ, de Pablo J. Response to 4-month treatment with reboxetine in Parkinson's disease patients with a major depressive episode. *Gen Hosp Psychiatry*. 2006;28:59-64.

65 Barone P, Scarzella L, Marconi R, et al; for the Depression/Parkinson Italian Study Group. Pramipexole versus sertraline in the treatment of depression in Parkinson's disease: a national multicenter parallel-group randomized study. *J Neurol*. 2006;253:601-607.

66 Levin OS. [Coaxil (tianeptine) in the treatment of depression in Parkinson's disease]. *Zh Nevrol Psikhiatr Im S S Korsakova*. 2006;106:20-25.

67   Kano O, Ikeda K, Kiyozuka T, et al. Beneficial effect of pramipexole for motor function and depression in Parkinson's disease. *Neuropsychiatr Dis Treat*. 2008;4:707-710.

68   Menza M, Dobkin RD, Marin H, et al A controlled trial of antidepressants in patients with Parkinson disease and depression. *Neurology*. 2009;72:886-892.

69   Werneck AL, Rosso AL, Vincent MB. The use of an antagonist 5-HT2a/c for depression and motor function in Parkinson' disease. *Arq Neuropsiquiatr*. 2009;67(2B):407-412.

70   Richard IH, McDermott MP, Kurlan R, et al; for the SAD-PD Study Group. A randomized, double-blind, placebo-controlled trial of antidepressants in Parkinson disease. *Neurology*. 2012;78:1229-1236.

71   Vu TC, Nutt JG, Holford NHG. Progression of motor and nonmotor features of Parkinson's disease and their response to treatment. *Br J Clin Pharmacol*. 2012;74:267-283.

72   Beck AT, Ward CH, Mendelson M, Mock J, Erbaugh J. An inventory for measuring depression. *Arch Gen Psychiatry*. 1961;4:561-571.

73   Beck AT, Steer RA, Ball R, Ranieri W. Comparison of Beck Depression Inventories -IA and -II in psychiatric outpatients. *J Pers Assess*. 1996;67:588-597.

74   Visser M, Leentjens AFG, Marinus J, et al. Reliability and validity of the Beck depression inventory in patients with Parkinson's disease. *Mov Disord*. 2006;21:668-672.

75   Levin BE, Llabre MM, Weiner WJ. Parkinson's disease and depression: psychometric properties of the Beck Depression Inventory. *J Neurol Neurosurg Psychiatry*. 1988;51:1401-1404.

76   Tumas V, Rodrigues GGR, Farias TLA, Crippa JAS. The accuracy of diagnosis of major depression in patients with Parkinson's disease: a comparative study among the UPDRS, the geriatric depression scale and the Beck depression inventory. *Arq Neuropsiquiatr*. 2008;66(2A):152-156.

77   Leentjens AF, Verhey FR, Luijckx GJ, Troost J. The validity of the Beck Depression Inventory as a screening and diagnostic instrument for depression in patients with Parkinson's disease. *Mov Disord*. 2000;15:1221-1224.

78   Silberman CD, Laks J, Capitão CF, Rodrigues CS, Moreira I, Engelhardt E. Recognizing depression in patients with Parkinson's disease: accuracy and specificity of two depression rating scale. *Arq Neuropsiquiatr*. 2006;64(2B):407-411.

79   Avila A, Cardona X, Martin-Baranera M, Maho P, Sastre F, Bello J. Does nefazodone improve both depression and Parkinson disease? A pilot randomized trial. *J Clin Psychopharmacol*. 2003;23:509-513.

80   Van Hemert DA, Van de Vijver FJR, Poortinga YH. The Beck Depression Inventory as a Measure of Subjective Well-Being: A Cross-National Study. *J Happiness Stud*. 2002;3:257-286.

81   Zigmond AS, Snaith RP. The hospital anxiety and depression scale. *Acta Psychiatr Scand*. 1983;67:361-370.

82   Marinus J, Leentjens AF, Visser M, Stiggelbout AM, van Hilten JJ. Evaluation of the hospital anxiety and depression scale in patients with Parkinson's disease. *Clin Neuropharmacol*. 2002;25:318-324.

83   Rodriguez-Blazquez C, Frades-Payo B, Forjaz MJ, de Pedro-Cuesta J, Martinez-Martin P; Longitudinal Parkinson's Disease Patient Study Group. Psychometric attributes of the Hospital Anxiety and Depression Scale in Parkinson's disease. *Mov Disord*. 2009;24:519-525.

84   Forjaz MJ, Rodriguez-Blázquez C, Martinez-Martin P. Rasch analysis of the hospital anxiety and depression scale in Parkinson's disease. *Mov Disord*. 2009;24:526-532.

85   Leentjens AF, Dujardin K, Marsh L, Richard IH, Starkstein SE, Martinez-Martin P. Anxiety rating scales in Parkinson's disease: a validation study of the Hamilton anxiety rating scale, the Beck anxiety inventory, and the hospital anxiety and depression scale. *Mov Disord*. 2011;26:407-415.

86   Mondolo F, Jahanshahi M, Granà A, Biasutti E, Cacciatori E, Di Benedetto P. Evaluation of anxiety in Parkinson's disease with some commonly used rating scales. *Neurol Sci*. 2007;28:270-275.

87   Martínez-Martín P, Valldeoriola F, Tolosa E, et al. Bilateral subthalamic nucleus stimulation and quality of life in advanced Parkinson's disease. *Mov Disord*. 2002;17:372-377.

88   Kulisevsky J, Pagonabarraga J, Pascual-Sedano B, Gironell A, García-Sánchez C, Martínez-Corral M. Motor changes during sertraline treatment in depressed patients with Parkinson's disease. *Eur J Neurol*. 2008;15:953-959.

89   Wade DT, Gage H, Owen C, Trend P, Grossmith C, Kaye J. Multidisciplinary rehabilitation for people with Parkinson's disease: a randomised controlled study. *J Neurol Neurosurg Psychiatry*. 2003;74:158-162.

90 Montgomery SA, Asberg M. A new depression scale designed to be sensitive to change. *Br J Psychiatry*. 1979;134:382-389.
91 Thommessen B, Aarsland D, Braekhus A, Oksengaard AR, Engedal K, Laake K. The psychosocial burden on spouses of the elderly with stroke, dementia and Parkinson's disease. *Int J Geriatr Psychiatry*. 2002;17:78-84.
92 Rektorova I, Balaz M, Svatova J, et al. Effects of ropinirole on nonmotor symptoms of Parkinson disease: a prospective multicenter study. *Clin Neuropharmacol*. 2008;31:261-266.
93 Montel S, Bonnet A-M, Bungener C. Quality of life in relation to mood, coping strategies, and dyskinesia in Parkinson's disease. *J Geriatr Psychiatry Neurol*. 2009;22:95-102.
94 Go CL, Rosales RL, Joya-Tanglao M, Fernandez HH. Untreated depressive symptoms among cognitively-intact, community dwelling Filipino patients with Parkinson disease. *Int J Neurosci*. 2011;121:137-141.
95 Riedel O, Dodel R, Deuschl G, et al. [Dementia and depression determine care dependency in Parkinson's disease: analysis of 1,449 outpatients receiving nursing care in Germany]. *Nervenarzt*. 2011;82:1012-1019.
96 Perez Lloret S, Rossi M, Merello M, Rascol O, Cardinali DP. Nonmotor symptoms groups in Parkinson's disease patients: results of a pilot, exploratory study. *Parkinsons Dis*. 2011;2011:473579.
97 Koerts J, Leenders KL, Koning M, Portman AT, van Beilen M. Striatal dopaminergic activity (FDOPA-PET) associated with cognitive items of a depression scale (MADRS) in Parkinson's disease. *Eur J Neurosci*. 2007;25:3132-3136.
98 Ehrt U, Larsen JP, Aarsland D. Pain and its relationship to depression in Parkinson disease. *Am J Geriatr Psychiatry*. 2009;17:269-275.
99 Riedel O, Heuser I, Klotsche J, Dodel R, Wittchen HU; GEPAD Study Group. Occurrence risk and structure of depression in Parkinson disease with and without dementia: results from the GEPAD Study. *J Geriatr Psychiatry Neurol*. 2010;23:27-34.
100 Riedel O, Dodel R, Deuschl G, et al. Depression and care-dependency in Parkinson's disease: results from a nationwide study of 1449 outpatients. *Parkinsonism Relat Disord*. 2012;18:598-601.
101 Arun MP, Bharath S, Pal PK, Singh G. Relationship of depression, disability, and quality of life in Parkinson's disease: a hospital-based case-control study. *Neurol India*. 2011;59:185-189.
102 Koerts J, Leenders KL, Koning M, Bouma A, van Beilen M. The assessment of depression in Parkinson's disease. *Eur J Neurol*. 2008;15:487-492.
103 Harada T, Ishizaki F, Horie N, et al. New dopamine agonist pramipexole improves parkinsonism and depression in Parkinson's disease. *Hiroshima J Med Sci*. 2011;60:79-82.
104 Da Silva TM, Munhoz RP, Alvarez C, et al. Depression in Parkinson's disease: a double-blind, randomized, placebo-controlled pilot study of omega-3 fatty-acid supplementation. *J Affect Disord*. 2008;111:351-359.
105 Mace JL, Porter RJ, Dalrymple-Alford JC, Anderson TJ. The effects of acute tryptophan depletion on mood in patients with Parkinson's disease and the healthy elderly. *J Psychopharmacol (Oxford)*. 2010;24:615-619.
106 Pal E, Nagy F, Aschermann Z, Balazs E, Kovacs N. The impact of left prefrontal repetitive transcranial magnetic stimulation on depression in Parkinson's disease: a randomized, double-blind, placebo-controlled study. *Mov Disord*. 2010;25:2311-2317.
107 Yesavage JA, Brink TL, Rose TL, et al. Development and validation of a geriatric depression screening scale: a preliminary report. *J Psychiatr Res*. 1982;17:37-49.
108 Sheikh JI, Yesavage JA. Geriatric Depression Scale (GDS): Recent evidence and development of a shorter version. Clinical Gerontologist: *Aging Ment Health*. 1986;5:165-173.
109 Montorio I, Izal M. The Geriatric Depression Scale: a review of its development and utility. *Int Psychogeriatr*. 1996;8:103-112.
110 Weintraub D, Oehlberg KA, Katz IR, Stern MB. Test Characteristics of the 15-Item Geriatric Depression Scale and Hamilton Depression Rating Scale in Parkinson Disease. *Am J Geriatr Psychiatry*. 2006;14:169-175.

111 Weintraub D, Xie S, Karlawish J, Siderowf A. Differences in depression symptoms in patients with Alzheimer's and Parkinson's diseases: evidence from the 15-item Geriatric Depression Scale (GDS-15). *Int J Geriatr Psychiatry*. 2007;22:1025-1030.

112 Ertan FS, Ertan T, Kiziltan G, Uyguçgil H. Reliability and validity of the Geriatric Depression Scale in depression in Parkinson's disease. *J Neurol Neurosurg Psychiatry*. 2005;76:1445-1447.

113 McDonald WM, Holtzheimer PE, Haber M, Vitek JL, McWhorter K, Delong M. Validity of the 30-item geriatric depression scale in patients with Parkinson's disease. *Mov Disord*. 2006;21:1618-1622.

114 Chagas MHN, Tumas V, Loureiro SR, et al. Validity of a Brazilian version of the Zung self-rating depression scale for screening of depression in patients with Parkinson's disease. *Parkinsonism Relat Disord*. 2010;16:42-45.

115 Meara J, Mitchelmore E, Hobson P. Use of the GDS-15 geriatric depression scale as a screening instrument for depressive symptomatology in patients with Parkinson's disease and their carers in the community. *Age Ageing*. 1999;28:35-38.

116 Weintraub D, Saboe K, Stern MB. Effect of age on Geriatric Depression Scale performance in Parkinson's Disease. *Mov Disord*. 2007;22:1331-1335.

117 Smania N, Corato E, Tinazzi M, et al. Effect of balance training on postural instability in patients with idiopathic Parkinson's disease. *Neurorehabil Neural Repair*. 2010;24:826-834.

118 Kum WF, Durairajan SSK, Bian ZX, et al. Treatment of idiopathic Parkinson's disease with traditional chinese herbal medicine: a randomized placebo-controlled pilot clinical study. *Evid Based Complement Alternat Med*. 2011;2011:724353.

119 Williams JR, Hirsch ES, Anderson K, et al. A comparison of nine scales to detect depression in Parkinson disease: which scale to use? *Neurology*. 2012;78:998-1006.

120 Thompson AW, Liu H, Hays RD, et al. Diagnostic accuracy and agreement across three depression assessment measures for Parkinson's disease. *Parkinsonism Relat Disord*. 2011;17:40-45.

121 Starkstein SE, Mayberg HS, Preziosi TJ, Andrezejewski P, Leiguarda R, Robinson RG. Reliability, validity, and clinical correlates of apathy in Parkinson's disease. *J Neuropsychiatry Clin Neurosci*. 1992;4:134-139.

122 Marin RS, Biedrzycki RC, Firinciogullari S. Reliability and validity of the Apathy Evaluation Scale. *Psychiatry Res*. 1991;38:143-162.

123 Starkstein SE, Ingram L, Garau ML, Mizrahi R. On the overlap between apathy and depression in dementia. *J Neurol Neurosurg Psychiatry*. 2005;76:1070-1074.

124 Pedersen KF, Alves G, Larsen JP, et al. Psychometric properties of the Starkstein Apathy Scale in patients with early untreated Parkinson disease. *Am J Geriatr Psychiatry*. 2012;20:142-148.

125 Zahodne LB, Young S, Kirsch-Darrow L, et al. Examination of the Lille Apathy Rating Scale in Parkinson disease. *Mov Disord*. 2009;24:677-683.

126 Czernecki V, Pillon B, Houeto JL, Pochon JB, Levy R, Dubois B. Motivation, reward, and Parkinson's disease: influence of dopatherapy. *Neuropsychologia*. 2002;40:2257-2267.

127 Czernecki V, Pillon B, Houeto JL, et al. Does bilateral stimulation of the subthalamic nucleus aggravate apathy in Parkinson's disease? *J Neurol Neurosurg Psychiatr*. 2005;76:775-779.

128 Drapier D, Drapier S, Sauleau P, et al. Does subthalamic nucleus stimulation induce apathy in Parkinson's disease? *J Neurol*. 2006;253:1083-1091.

129 Funkiewiez A, Ardouin C, Cools R, et al. Effects of levodopa and subthalamic nucleus stimulation on cognitive and affective functioning in Parkinson's disease. *Mov Disord*. 2006;21:1656-1662.

8. Quality of life scales

The most commonly used quality of life scales purposely developed for Parkinson's disease (PD) are described in this chapter. In addition, two generic scales that cover relevant health domains for PD are also presented.

Parkinson's Disease Questionnaire (PDQ) 39 items (PDQ-39) [1] 8 items (PDQ-8) [2]	
Description of scale	
Overview	These questionnaires assess subjective health status [1], although they are classified as health-related quality of life instruments [3]. PDQ-39 is composed of 39 items grouped into 8 subscales
	PDQ-8 is the short version of the PDQ-39, with eight items each representing a PDQ-39 domain. For both scales, responses are scored in a Likert-type scale from 0 (never) to 4 (always). Subscale scores are transformed into a 0-100 scale by summing the items' raw scores, dividing them by the maximum possible raw score, and then multiplying by 100. A Summary Index (SI) is also calculated. Higher scores mean lower quality of life
	Time to complete the scale: 15 minutes for completing the PDQ-39
	Time frame: the month prior to assessment
	Self-administered by interview and by proxy evaluations have been also tested [4]
	Specific for patients with PD
Copyright?	Owned by Isis Innovation Limited
How can the scale be obtained?	For obtaining the scales, the manual, and the license: University of Oxford (Isis Innovation Limited) www.publichealth.ox.ac.uk/units/hsru/PDQ/
	www.isis-innovation.com/licensing/healthoutcomes/
Clinimetric properties of scale in patients with PD	
Feasibility	Older people and those with more severe impairments could have difficulties with the response options, and could perceive some PDQ-39 items as not relevant and the questionnaire as too long [5]. PDQ-8 is intended to address some of these issues [3]
Dimensionality	PDQ-39 appears to be multidimensional but its structure has not been well established [6]. For PDQ-8, factor analysis has identified a single factor [7]
Acceptability	Observed range scores were almost coincident with the possible range for both scales. No floor or ceiling effects were detected [3]

© Springer Healthcare 2014
P. Martinez-Martin et al., *Guide to Assessment Scales in Parkinson's Disease*,
DOI: 10.1007/978-1-907673-88-7_8

Reliability	Internal consistency: satisfactory for PDQ-39 (Cronbach's alpha: 0.84 to 0.97), although some items in the Stigma, Social Support, Cognitions, Communication, and Bodily Discomfort domains showed lower item-total correlation [1,8]. PDQ-8 internal consistency was also suitable, with lower indices than PDQ-39 [3]
	Inter-rater and test-retest reliability: appropriate for both scales [3,9]
Validity	Content validity: reported as satisfactory for PDQ-39, although it lacks some relevant areas [3]. Not tested for PDQ-8
	Convergent: close correlations of with other quality of life and clinical scales [3,9]
	Known-groups: significant differences by Hoehn & Yahr Staging Scale (HY) stages [1,2,9]
	Internal: inter-domain correlations between 0.09 to 0.71 in the case of PDQ-39 [8]
	Predictive: PDQ-39 can predict EQ-5D, Schedule for the Evaluation of Individual Quality of Life (SEIQOL), and some non-motor symptoms [10,11]
Responsiveness & Interpretability	PDQ-39 and PDQ-8 have been widely applied as an outcome measure in clinical trials, and have been proved to be sensitive to changes in health status [3,12,13]
	Minimal important difference (MID) has been calculated for both scales [14,15]
	Both scales are applicable in patients with PD of both sexes and at all ages. However, some PDQ-39 items showed differential item functioning (DIF) by sex and age [6] and older people and those with more impairments can have difficulties completing the questionnaire [5]
Cross-cultural Adaptations & Others	Both scales are available in several languages and have been used in different cultural settings [3]
Overall impression	
Advantages	Includes dimensions relevant to patients with PD; widely used and extensively analyzed across different settings and countries; adequate psychometric properties; responsive to changes. PDQ-8 retains the satisfactory properties of the PDQ-39 and provides similar information. Both scales are recommended by the Movement Disorder Society (MDS)-Task force [3]
Disadvantages	They lack some relevant areas for PD; some limitations in reliability; dimensionality not well established; for PDQ-8, some clinimetric properties need further analysis

Parkinson's Disease quality of life questionnaire (PDQL) [16]	
Description of scale	
Overview	The PDQL measures quality of life in patients with PD
	It is made up of 37 items, grouped into four domains: Parkinsonian (14 items) and Systemic (7) symptoms; and Social (7) and Emotional (9) function. Items are scored form 1 to 5, and the total score is obtained by summing the item scores (higher scores indicate better quality of life)
	Time to complete the scale is 23 ± 2.7 minutes [17]
	Self-administered questionnaire, although it may also be administered by interview [18]
	This scale was specifically developed for and validated in patients with PD
Copyright?	The scale is published in the original publication, but permission from the authors is required for its use [16]
How can the scale be obtained?	Distribution of the scale is done through MAPI: www.mapi-trust.org/services/questionnairelicensing/catalog-questionnaires
Clinimetric properties of scale in patients with PD	
Feasibility	Questions are appropriate for PD. The PDQL is potentially applicable across all PD states, except for patients with significant cognitive impairment [16]
Dimensionality	Multidimensional scale. Dimensions were defined according to exploratory factor analysis [16]. Other studies did not explore the factor structure of the PDQL
Acceptability	No floor or ceiling effect; skewness within standard limits [8,17,19]
Reliability	Internal consistency: high for the summary index (>0.90) and mostly adequate for the domains (≥0.65) [8,17,19,20]
	Test-retest reliability: no significant differences between two applications over two weeks [19]; adequate intra-class correlation coefficients and kappa values for a seven-day comparison [8]
Validity	Adequate face validity [9] for PD population
	Moderate-to-high convergent validity with other quality of life scales and related-construct measures such as HY, disability scales and depression [8,16,17,19,20]. The PDQL showed significant differences by HY stage, and Schwab & England Activities of Daily Living Scale (SE), and Webster levels [8,16,19–21]
	Satisfactory internal validity [8]
Responsiveness & Interpretability	Sensitive to change by exercise therapy [22], unilateral pallidotomy and bilateral subthalamic nucleus stimulation [23–27]. In 12-month follow-up studies, most PDQL scores showed significant changes [28], although with small effect sizes [13,28]. Standardized response mean ranged from 6.31 to 7.80 [8,13,20]
	There is no information about minimal clinical difference
Cross-cultural Adaptations & Others	The scale is available in several languages such as English, Dutch, French, German, Italian, Portuguese, and Spanish. There are formal validations for the Spanish [8,17], Dutch [16], and Portuguese versions [19]

Overall impression	
Advantages	'Recommended' for use in PD by the MDS-Task Force [3]; possesses sound clinimetric properties; widely used
Disadvantages	Some quality of life areas are covered in less depth than the PDQ-38 [9]

Scales for Outcomes in Parkinson's Disease -Psychosocial (SCOPA-PS) [29]	
Description of scale	
Overview	Assesses psychosocial functioning in patients with PD [29]
	The SCOPA-PS is composed of 11 items representing social or emotional consequences of PD, scored from 0 (not at all) to 3 (very much). Higher scores reflect greater psychosocial difficulties
	Time to complete the scale: not calculated
	Time frame: the month prior to assessment
	Rater: the patient
	Specific for PD
Copyright?	Public domain
How can the scale be obtained?	The scale can be obtained free of charge from the SCOPA website: www.scopa-propark.eu
Clinimetric properties of scale in patients with PD	
Feasibility	SCOPA-PS has been used for patients with PD of all levels of severity and with a broad range of disease duration [29,30]
Dimensionality	Uncertain: studies have identified a one- or two-factor structure [3,30,31]
Acceptability	Item on sexual problems frequently presents missing values. No skewness, floor or ceiling effects [29–31]
Reliability	Internal consistency and item-total correlations are satisfactory as a whole [29–33]
	Inter-rater reliability: not tested
	Test-retest reliability: satisfactory [29,32]
Validity	Content validity satisfactory [31]. Items were generated based on review of literature. Item reduction phase was performed in a pilot study [29]. It lacks questions on physical and mental domains
	Convergent: high correlation coefficients with PDQ-39, EQ-5D, Clinical Impression of Severity Index for Parkinson's Disease (CISI-PD) and Hospital Anxiety and Depression Scale (HADS), moderate with Medical Outcomes Study-Short Form 36 (SF-36) and HY [29–33]
	Known-groups: SCOPA-PS scores increased with PD severity levels [30,31]

Responsiveness & Interpretability	Standard error of measurement (SEM) has been determined [30,31,33]
	Minimally important change: 8.30 to 9.10 points. Threshold value for a significant change (smallest real difference and reliable change index) and threshold values for a clinically meaningful change (effect size, standardized response mean, responsiveness statistic) were calculated [33]. Change in SCOPA-PS scores correlated strongly with change in total Unified Parkinson's Disease Rating Scale (UPDRS), HADS, and PDQ-39 scores, and reliably detected 70% of cases that worsened according to the PDQ-39 [33]
	No significant differences in SCOPA-PS between men and women [29,30]
	Item on sexuality can be problematic for older people
Cross-cultural Adaptations & Others	The scale has been validated in the Netherlands, Brazil, Argentina, Ecuador, Paraguay, and Spain [29–32]
Overall impression	
Advantages	Short and easy questionnaire; sound clinimetric properties; valid and reliable in different languages; 'recommended' scale by the MDS [3]
Disadvantages	Evaluates only psychosocial functioning and does not cover all domains of quality of life a high percentage of missing values for the item addressing sexual problems

Parkinson's Impact Scale (PIMS) [34]	
Description of scale	
Overview	The PIMS measures the impact of Parkinson's disease on the patient's emotional, social, and economic life [34], or the patient's quality of life [35]. It is formed by ten items scored in a five-point response scale (from 0=no change, to 4=severe), and a higher total score indicates more impact on PD
	Time frame: No time frame is specified
	Time to complete the scale: less than ten minutes [34]
	Rated by the patient or the caregiver [36]
	This is a specific scale for PD
Copyright?	The scale was published as an erratum to the original publication [37]
How can the scale be obtained?	
Clinimetric properties of scale in patients with PD	
Feasibility	Appropriate for PD population. However, significant cognitive impairment compromises the scale's self-administration
Dimensionality	Exploratory factor analysis indentified four factors: Psychological, Social, Physical, and Financial [34]
Acceptability	Good data quality except for item on sexuality; no floor or ceiling effects and skewness within the standard limits [17]
Reliability	Internal consistency: high (0.87 to 0.90) [17,34,35]
	Adequate test-retest reliability (intraclass correlation coefficient: 0.72 to 0.98) [17,34,35]
	No information on inter-rater reliability

Validity	Content validity is satisfactory as a whole, although it was criticized for lacking items related to physical and mental aspects [9]
	Adequate convergent validity with HADS, UPDRS, and disability measures, as well other PD quality of life measures (PDQ-39 and PDQL) [17]
	Established know-groups validity by HY stage and fluctuations [17,34,38]
	Moderate and high correlations with the rating scale for gait evaluation [39] and the Parkinson's disease symptom inventory [40], respectively
Responsiveness & Interpretability	Adequate sensitivity to change in a cross-over trial of tolcapone [35]. No information on minimal important difference
Cross-cultural adaptations & Others	There are studies reporting the PIMS application in India, Canada, and Ecuador. The bilingual Canadian and Ecuador versions have been formally validated [17,35]
Overall impression	
Advantages	'Recommended' scale for quality of life in PD [3]; very short quality of life scale; sound clinimetric properties
Disadvantages	Limited information on responsiveness and interpretability; lacks information on physical and mental aspects of PD

EQ-5D [41]	
Description of scale	
Overview	Assesses health status [41], although it is classified as a quality of life measure [3]
	Composed of 5 item-domains (mobility, self-care, usual activities, pain/discomfort, and anxiety/depression), each with 3 possible responses, scored from 1 (no problems) to 3 (severe problems). It provides a profile for the individual (eg, 11211), and can be translated into health scores (from 0=worst possible health, to 1=perfect health) for cost-utility analysis. Additionally, a visual analogue scale (VAS) assesses the self-rated global 'health state today' on a vertical bar running from 100 ('best imaginable health state') to 0 ('worst imaginable health state')
	Time to complete the scale: ten minutes
	Time frame: day of assessment
	Rater: self-administered. By proxy and by interview formats have been tested [4]
	Generic, but successfully validated and applied in patients with PD [3,42,43]
Copyright?	The EQ-5D is owned by the EuroQol Group
How can the scale be obtained?	Information about how to obtain the EQ-5D is available on the website: www.euroqol.org
Clinimetric properties of scale in patients with PD	
Feasibility	It covers relevant health domains for PD and can be used across all PD stages [42], but may be insensitive in mild PD and in patients with motor complications [44]
Dimensionality	Multidimensional, but its structure has not been tested in PD

Acceptability	Low rate of missing responses [42]
	Score distribution: mean (SD) of 0.62–0.73 (0.26) [42,43] for EQ-5D index
	Skewness and floor and ceiling effects not reported in PD
Reliability	Inter-rater reliability: satisfactory patient vs. caregivers agreement for the EQ-5D index, but not for three items of the descriptive system [4]
Validity	Content validity: not formally tested, although it is deemed to cover relevant health domains for PD [42]
	Convergent: strong correlations with other generic and specific quality of life scales (PDQ-39/8, SF-36, etc.) and clinical scales (Beck Depression Inventory [BDI], SE). Low-to-moderate correlations with HY, UPDRS, and Mini Mental State Examination (MMSE) [42,43]
	Known-groups: significant differences in EQ-5D index by depression severity (BDI), cognitive status (MMSE), motor impairment (UPDRS), and HY stages [42,44]
Responsiveness & Interpretability	Used in clinical trials, EQ-5D can capture changes in health status over time [3]. The index is more sensitive than the VAS [45]. However, the EQ-5D did not show changes in a one-year longitudinal study [28], suggesting that it is best utilized to capture large changes in quality of life
	Some responsiveness indices have been calculated [13,45]
	No significant differences by sex or age in patients with PD [42]
Cross-cultural Adaptations & Others	Translated into several languages. Normative data for the general population are also available (www.euroqol.org)
Overall impression	
Advantages	Allows comparisons with other medical conditions; sound clinimetric properties in patients with PD; widely used as an outcome measure; useful for econometric studies; 'recommended' by the MDS [3]
Disadvantages	Some clinimetric properties have not been analyzed in PD; only partially responsive over time

Medical Outcomes Study-Short Form 36 (SF-36) [46].	
Description of scale	
Overview	Assesses health status [46], although it has been labeled as a quality of life measure [3]
	It consists of 36 questions and gives scores in eight different domains. Summary scores for physical and mental function can be calculated. A score between 0 and 100 can be calculated for each domain, as well as for the summary scales, with higher scores representing better health status. Items are scored in a yes/no format and in a five-point scale
	Time to complete the scale: 5 to 10 minutes [47]
	Time frame: 4 week period prior to assessment
	Self-rated. Administration by interview has been also tried [48]
	Generic, although validated for PD [3]

Copyright?	Copyright of QualityMetric Incorporated
How can the scale be obtained?	www.sf-36.org/tools/sf36.shtml
Clinimetric properties of scale in patients with PD	
Feasibility	Some relevant areas in PD are not included and some questions may not be suitable for patients with PD [49–51]
Dimensionality	Multidimensional, but findings do not support the use of physical and mental scores in PD [51,52]
Acceptability	Missing data and floor and ceiling effects were present in some domains, particularly in older patients [53,54]. Administration by interview and an amended version did not overcome this problem [48]
Reliability	Internal consistency: satisfactory, as a whole, for subscales and total score [54]
	Inter-rater reliability: not tested
	Test-retest reliability: satisfactory, as a whole [51,55]
Validity	Content validity: adequate; some PD-relevant areas are not covered [48,56]
	Convergent: high correlation coefficients with other generic and specific quality of life scales (PDQ-39, EQ-5D) and clinical measures [9,56,57]
	Known-groups: SF-36 can discriminate between groups of patients based on disease severity, comorbidity, and disability [49,53,56]
Responsiveness & Interpretability	Yes. It has been used as an outcome measure in clinical trials, and it is more responsive than other PD-specific measures [13,49]
	The minimally detectable change (MDC) (IC 95%) values for the SF-36 ranged between 19% and 45% [55]
	Missing responses are more likely in older patients with PD [53,54]
Cross-cultural Adaptations & Others	Translated and validated into several languages. An improved version for older patients has been tested [48]
Overall impression	
Advantages	Short; reliable; valid and responsive in patients with PD; 'recommended' by the MDS [3]
Disadvantages	Some flaws in feasibility and acceptability; two-domain structure not supported in patients with PD

Figure 8.1 Scales for Outcomes in Parkinson's disease–PsychoSocial (SCOPA-PS)

In this questionnaire, we inquire about problems which you may encounter as a result of your illness in the areas of (social) activities, contact with other people, and on an emotional level. When answering the following questions, please think carefully about your personal situation during the _past month_, and consider to what extent the situation described actually posed a problem for you. Tick the box next to the answer which best reflects your situation.

1   During the past month, have you had difficulty with work, household or other chores?
☐ not at all   ☐ a little   ☐ quite a bit   ☐ very much

2   During the past month, have you had difficulty with hobbies, sport or leisure activities?
☐ not at all   ☐ a little   ☐ quite a bit   ☐ very much

3 During the past month, have you felt uncertain in your contact with others?
☐ not at all ☐ a little ☐ quite a bit ☐ very much

4 During the past month, have you had problems getting along with your partner, family, or good friends?
☐ not at all ☐ a little ☐ quite a bit ☐ very much

5 During the past month, have you had problems in the area of sexuality?
☐ not at all ☐ a little ☐ quite a bit ☐ very much

6 During the past month, have you felt more house-bound than you would wish to be?
☐ not at all ☐ a little ☐ quite a bit ☐ very much

7 To what extent have you had the feeling that you have had to ask others for help too often during the past month?
☐ not at all ☐ a little ☐ quite a bit ☐ very much

8 To what extent have you felt isolated and lonely during the past month?
☐ not at all ☐ a little ☐ quite a bit ☐ very much

9 During the past month, have you had difficulty when having a conversation?
☐ not at all ☐ a little ☐ quite a bit ☐ very much

10 To what extent have you felt ashamed of your disease during the past month?
☐ not at all ☐ a little ☐ quite a bit ☐ very much

11 During the past month, have you been concerned about the future?
☐ not at all ☐ a little ☐ quite a bit ☐ very much

References

1 Peto V, Jenkinson C, Fitzpatrick R, Greenhall R. The development and validation of a short measure of functioning and well being for individuals with Parkinson's disease. *Qual Life Res*. 1995;4:241-248.
2 Jenkinson C, Fitzpatrick R, Peto V, et al. The PDQ-8: Development and validation of a short-form parkinson's disease questionnaire. *Psychol Health*. 1997;12:805-814.
3 Martinez-Martin P, Jeukens-Visser M, Lyons KE, et al. Health-related quality-of-life scales in Parkinson's disease: critique and recommendations. *Mov Disord*. 2011;26:2371-2380.
4 Martínez-Martín P, Benito-León J, Alonso F, Catalán MJ, Pondal M, Zamarbide I. Health-related quality of life evaluation by proxy in Parkinson's disease: approach using PDQ-8 and EuroQoL-5D. *Mov Disord*. 2004;19:312-318.
5 Hagell P. Feasibility and linguistic validity of the Swedish version of the PDQ-39. *Expert Rev Pharmacoecon Outcomes Res*. 2005;5:131-136.
6 Hagell P, Nygren C. The 39 item Parkinson's disease questionnaire (PDQ-39) revisited: implications for evidence based medicine. *J Neurol Neurosurg Psychiatr*. 2007;78:1191-1198.
7 Jenkinson C, Fitzpatrick R. Cross-cultural evaluation of the short form 8-item Parkinson's Disease Questionnaire (PDQ-8): results from America, Canada, Japan, Italy and Spain. *Parkinsonism Relat Disord*. 2007;13:22-28.
8 Martinez-Martin P, Serrano-Dueñas M, Forjaz MJ, Serrano MS. Two questionnaires for Parkinson's disease: are the PDQ-39 and PDQL equivalent? *Qual Life Res*. 2007;16:1221-1230.

9 Marinus J, Ramaker C, Van Hilten JJ, Stiggelbout AM. Health related quality of life in Parkinson's disease: a systematic review of disease specific instruments. *J Neurol Neurosurg Psychiatr.* 2002;72:241-248.

10 Grosset D, Taurah L, Burn DJ, et al. A multicentre longitudinal observational study of changes in self reported health status in people with Parkinson's disease left untreated at diagnosis. *J Neurol Neurosurg Psychiatr.* 2007;78:465-469.

11 Young MK, Ng S-K, Mellick G, Scuffham PA. Mapping of the PDQ-39 to EQ-5D scores in patients with Parkinson's disease? *Qual Life Res.* 2013;22:1065-1072.

12 Martinez-Martin P, Deuschl G. Effect of medical and surgical interventions on health-related quality of life in Parkinson's disease. *Mov Disord.* 2007;22:757-765.

13 Schrag A, Spottke A, Quinn NP, Dodel R. Comparative responsiveness of Parkinson's disease scales to change over time. *Mov Disord.* 2009;24:813-818.

14 Peto V, Jenkinson C, Fitzpatrick R. Determining minimally important differences for the PDQ-39 Parkinson's disease questionnaire. *Age Ageing.* 2001;30:299-302.

15 Luo N, Tan LC, Zhao Y, Lau PN, Au WL, Li SC. Determination of the longitudinal validity and minimally important difference of the 8-item Parkinson's Disease Questionnaire (PDQ-8). *Mov Disord.* 2009;24:183-187.

16 De Boer AG, Wijker W, Speelman JD, De Haes JC. Quality of life in patients with Parkinson's disease: development of a questionnaire. *J Neurol Neurosurg Psychiatr.* 1996;61:70-74.

17 Serrano-Dueñas M, Serrano S. Psychometric characteristics of PIMS--compared to PDQ-39 and PDQL- -to evaluate quality of life in Parkinson's disease patients: validation in Spanish (Ecuadorian style). *Parkinsonism Relat Disord.* 2008;14:126-132.

18 Damiano AM, Snyder C, Strausser B, Willian MK. A review of health-related quality-of-life concepts and measures for Parkinson's disease. *Qual Life Res.* 1999;8:235-243.

19 Campos M, de Rezende CH, Farnese Vda C, da Silva CH, Morales NM, Pinto Rde M. Translation, cross-cultural adaptation, and validation of the Parkinson's Disease Quality of Life Questionnaire (PDQL), the "PDQL-BR", into Brazilian Portuguese. *ISRN Neurol.* 2011;2011:954787.

20 Serrano-Dueñas M, Martínez-Martín P, Vaca-Baquero V. Validation and cross-cultural adjustment of PDQL-questionnaire, Spanish version (Ecuador) (PDQL-EV). *Parkinsonism Relat Disord.* 2004;10:433-437.

21 Hobson P, Holden A, Meara J. Measuring the impact of Parkinson's disease with the Parkinson's Disease Quality of Life questionnaire. *Age Ageing.* 1999;28:341-346.

22 Yousefi B, Tadibi V, Khoei AF, Montazeri A. Exercise therapy, quality of life, and activities of daily living in patients with Parkinson disease: a small scale quasi-randomised trial. *Trials.* 2009;10:67.

23 De Bie RM, De Haan RJ, Nijssen PC, et al. Unilateral pallidotomy in Parkinson's disease: a randomised, single-blind, multicentre trial. *Lancet.* 1999;354:1665-1669.

24 de Bie RM, Schuurman PR, Bosch DA, de Haan RJ, Schmand B, Speelman JD; Dutch Pallidotomy Study Group. Outcome of unilateral pallidotomy in advanced Parkinson's disease: cohort study of 32 patients. *J Neurol Neurosurg Psychiatr.* 2001;71:375-382.

25 Esselink RAJ, De Bie RMA, De Haan RJ, et al. Unilateral pallidotomy versus bilateral subthalamic nucleus stimulation in PD: a randomized trial. *Neurology.* 2004;62:201-207.

26 Fraix V, Houeto J-L, Lagrange C, et al. Clinical and economic results of bilateral subthalamic nucleus stimulation in Parkinson's disease. *J Neurol Neurosurg Psychiatry.* 2006;77:443-449.

27 Lagrange E, Krack P, Moro E, Ardouin C, et al. Bilateral subthalamic nucleus stimulation improves health-related quality of life in PD. *Neurology.* 2002;59:1976-1978.

28 Reuther M, Spottke EA, Klotsche J, et al. Assessing health-related quality of life in patients with Parkinson's disease in a prospective longitudinal study. *Parkinsonism Relat Disord.* 2007;13:108-114.

29 Marinus J, Visser M, Martínez-Martín P, Van Hilten JJ, Stiggelbout AM. A short psychosocial questionnaire for patients with Parkinson's disease: the SCOPA-PS. *J Clin Epidemiol.* 2003;56:61-67.

30 Martínez-Martín P, Carroza-García E, Frades-Payo B, et al; for the Grupo ELEP. [Psychometric attributes of the Scales for Outcomes in Parkinson's Disease-Psychosocial (SCOPA-PS): validation in Spain and review]. *Rev Neurol.* 2009;49:1-7.

31 Virués-Ortega J, Carod-Artal FJ, Serrano-Dueñas M, et al. Cross-cultural validation of the Scales for Outcomes in Parkinson's Disease-Psychosocial questionnaire (SCOPA-PS) in four Latin American countries. *Value Health* 2009;12:385-391.

32 Carod-Artal FJ, Martinez-Martin P, Vargas AP. Independent validation of SCOPA-psychosocial and metric properties of the PDQ-39 Brazilian version. *Mov Disord*. 2007;22:91-98.

33 Martínez-Martin P, Carod-Artal FJ, da Silveira Ribeiro L, et al. Longitudinal psychometric attributes, responsiveness, and importance of change: An approach using the SCOPA-Psychosocial questionnaire. *Mov Disord*. 2008;23:1516-1523.

34 Calne S, Schulzer M, Mak E, et al. Validating a quality of life rating scale for idiopathic parkinsonism: Parkinson's Impact Scale (PIMS). *Parkinsonism Relat Disord*. 1996;2:55-61.

35 Schulzer M, Mak E, Calne SM. The psychometric properties of the Parkinson's Impact Scale (PIMS) as a measure of quality of life in Parkinson's disease. *Parkinsonism Relat Disord*. 2003;9:291-294.

36 Calne SM, Mak E, Hall J, et al. Validating a quality-of-life scale in caregivers of patients with Parkinson's disease: Parkinson's Impact Scale (PIMS). *Adv Neurol*. 2003;91:115-122.

37 Calne S, Schulzer M, Guyette C, et al. Erratum: Parkinson's Impact Scale. *Parkinsonism Relat Disord*. 1996;2:237.

38 Ray J, Das SK, Gangopadhya PK, Roy T. Quality of life in Parkinson's disease--Indian scenario. *J Assoc Physicians India*. 2006;54:17-21.

39 Serrano-Dueñas M, Calero B, Serrano S, Serrano M, Coronel P. Psychometric attributes of the rating scale for gait evaluation in Parkinson's disease. *Mov Disord*. 2010;25:2121-2127.

40 Hogan T, Grimaldi R, Dingemanse J, Martin M, Lyons K, Koller W. The Parkinson's disease symptom inventory (PDSI): a comprehensive and sensitive instrument to measure disease symptoms and treatment side-effects. *Parkinsonism Relat Disord*. 1999;5:93-98.

41 The EuroQol Group. EuroQol–a new facility for the measurement of health-related quality of life. The EuroQol Group. *1990*;16:199-208.

42 Schrag A, Selai C, Jahanshahi M, Quinn NP. The EQ-5D--a generic quality of life measure-is a useful instrument to measure quality of life in patients with Parkinson's disease. *J Neurol Neurosurg Psychiatry*. 2000;69:67-73.

43 Luo N, Low S, Lau PN, Au WL, Tan LC. Is EQ-5D a valid quality of life instrument in patients with Parkinson's disease? A study in Singapore. *Ann Acad Med Singap ore*. 2009;38:521-528.

44 Siderowf A, Ravina B, Glick HA. Preference-based quality-of-life in patients with Parkinson's disease. *Neurology*. 2002;59:103-108.

45 Luo N, Ng WY, Lau PN, Au WL, Tan LC. Responsiveness of the EQ-5D and 8-item Parkinson's Disease Questionnaire (PDQ-8) in a 4-year follow-up study. *Qual Life Res*. 2010;19:565-569.

46 Ware JE Jr, Sherbourne CD. The MOS 36-item short-form health survey (SF-36). I. Conceptual framework and item selection. *Med Care*. 1992;30:473-483.

47 McHorney CA, Ware JE Jr, Raczek AE. The MOS 36-Item Short-Form Health Survey (SF-36): II. Psychometric and clinical tests of validity in measuring physical and mental health constructs. *Med Care*. 1993;31:247-263.

48 Kuopio AM, Marttila RJ, Helenius H, Toivonen M, Rinne UK. The quality of life in Parkinson's disease. *Mov Disord*. 2000;15:216-223.

49 Brown CA, Cheng EM, Hays RD, Vassar SD, Vickrey BG. SF-36 includes less Parkinson Disease (PD)-targeted content but is more responsive to change than two PD-targeted health-related quality of life measures. *Qual Life Res*. 2009;18:1219-1237.

50 Hagell P, Reimer J, Nyberg P. Whose quality of life? Ethical implications in patient-reported health outcome measurement. *Value Health*. 2009;12:613-617.

51 Hagell P, Törnqvist AL, Hobart J. Testing the SF-36 in Parkinson's disease. Implications for reporting rating scale data. *J Neurol*. 2008;255:246-254.

52 Banks P, Martin CR. The factor structure of the SF-36 in Parkinson's disease. *J Eval Clin Pract*. 2009;15:460-463.

53 Hobson JP, Meara RJ. Is the SF-36 health survey questionnaire suitable as a self-report measure of the health status of older adults with Parkinson's disease? *Qual Life Res.* 1997;6:213-216.

54 Den Oudsten BL, Van Heck GL, De Vries J. The suitability of patient-based measures in the field of Parkinson's disease: a systematic review. *Mov Disord.* 2007;22:1390-1401.

55 Steffen T, Seney M. Test-retest reliability and minimal detectable change on balance and ambulation tests, the 36-item short-form health survey, and the unified Parkinson disease rating scale in people with parkinsonism. *Phys Ther.* 2008;88:733-746.

56 Jenkinson C, Peto V, Fitzpatrick R, Greenhall R, Hyman N. Self-reported functioning and well-being in patients with Parkinson's disease: comparison of the short-form health survey (SF-36) and the Parkinson's Disease Questionnaire (PDQ-39). *Age Ageing.* 1995;24:505-509.

57 Martínez Martín P, Frades B, Jiménez Jiménez FJ, et al. The PDQ-39 Spanish version: reliability and correlation with the short-form health survey (SF-36). *Neurologia.* 1999;14:159-163.